Red Road to Sinai is an honest account of Cate's journey
from a happy child, launched from a loving family,
to a woman trapped in a web of domestic violence.
Violence so insidious that it enlisted the mental health
and family court systems to completely destroy
Cate's sense of self, worth and purpose.

However, throughout Cate's story we see the back story
of God working miracles, sending messengers and sending
signs to prepare Cate for the most exciting part of her journey:
becoming the woman she was meant to be.

Cate's story is unique to her lived experience but also well outlines
the telltale tactics of violence and control used by an abusive partner.

Cate's brave writing style also shows the mental and emotional
anguish endured by domestic violence victims, most often women,
as they try to make sense out of lies and fabrications
being told to them by the person they love and trust the most.

Kim Olden M.Ed., LPC-S

Kim Olden is a Licensed Professional Counselor in Texas and the Chief Programs Officer at Hill Country Crisis Council, a Family Violence/ Sexual Assault Center serving the Texas Hill Country. Kim holds a master's degree in educational counseling from Sul Ross University and has 32 years of experience providing services to survivors of physical abuse, sexual abuse, family violence and sexual assault.

Red Sea Road to Sinai

For book reviews & more: **www.RedSeaRoadToSiani.com**

Yehovah is my light and my deliverance;
Whom should I fear?
Yehovah is the refuge of my life;
Whom should I dread?

Psalm 27:1

Great Publishing Company
Benai Emunah Institute
Kerrville, Texas

ISBN: 978-1-957488-13-4

Cover Artwork: Lisa Townley - **LoveWinsFineArt.com**
All Scripture quotations are from the
New King James Bible, unless otherwise noted.

Words from Dr. Miles Jones

Cate Jones is an accomplished author in her home country of New Zealand. In her latest book, ***Red Sea Road to Sinai***, her skill as a writer has transformed *her* journey into *our* journey.

Most of us have faced difficult and painful, even life-threatening circumstances. Some are presently facing circumstances that will either make or break them! For those who are in a desperate struggle for survival and sanity, this book offers great hope and spiritual help.

Cate shares her journey of *faith and courage* – a journey to *freedom and healing* - and a very real journey to the *Mount Sinai* of the Bible!

This true story is a unique revelation of a medical establishment that is supposed to heal us but is often incompetent, sometimes even evil in its harm and greed. So too, the modern mental health industry is crumbling before our eyes yet still making enormous amounts of money. This story is also about the Christian Church, that is often clueless in its response to the most prevalent problems people face in society today. Not only have our wider communities seen a massive increase in issues such as mental, physical and sexual abuse, but these have now become rampant in Christian marriages. Although Cate encountered many extraordinary individuals living out their faith by helping others heal, the Church is often asleep at the wheel. To survive the "*solutions*" offered by doctors and churchmen, a full-on encounter with The Savior is required to find ultimate freedom, healing and transformation. Cate testifies to this.

I have been deeply moved and deeply shaken by Cate's words. My great admiration for Cate - what she has endured, what she has overcome, and the remarkable woman of spiritual healing she has become - has led me to deeper faith and trust in Yehovah. **This is a guidebook for finding faith and healing in the most difficult of circumstances.**

It is a remarkable book in so many ways.

The obvious, is our climactic marriage at Mount Sinai, and the miracles that accompanied the Ketubah marriage ceremony. This was the same ceremony of the Israelites, 3500 years ago!

This was beyond my ability to explain. Cate has done a much better job than I in expressing the depth of this incredible emotional and spiritual experience. For me, it is the story of marrying my beloved wife Cate - in the most momentous way possible - at Moses' altar with Mount Sinai looming above us. To Cate it was a rich tapestry of emotional and spiritual realizations – put into words!

This is a book for *Overcomers*, or how to become one! If you want to see the power of God in action, ***Red Sea Road to Sinai*** is for you!

Dr. Miles R Jones

Contents

The Exodus

Acknowledgements

For I am not ashamed of the gospel,
because it is the power of God that brings salvation
to everyone who believes: first to the Jew, then to the Gentile.
Romans 1:16

I first and foremost lift up The Name of The One who has lifted me up, time and time again, Yehovah-Yeshua, my God and King. **You** have turned, and are still turning, every test and trial of my life into a testimony! **There is no other name under Heaven or on Earth, by which I could ever have been saved!**

To my husband Miles, who entered my story and is now walking out this journey with me. I am deeply grateful that you helped me get started on this book. Then to weather the many *emotional storms* that came, when the psychological hurdles of writing this story seemed too difficult for me to get over. Your love and persistent belief in me and my writing ability, got me to the finish-line. Thank you. I love you.

With immense gratitude to Kim Olden, Lindsey Erwin, and Lisa Townley, who assisted me significantly on the USA side of my life with: trauma therapy, friendship, counsel, and prayer ministry - *respectively*. You have each been a *tremendous* help and blessing. I love you all. Additional thanks to Lisa Townley, for your wonderful artwork on the cover!

To Rae Lloyd-Jones, Chief-Editor extraordinaire…you did a brilliant job of helping polish this story, or *"gem"* as you call it! Thank you too for encouraging me to write this book - affirming its value and need. You are a treasured sister-friend indeed!

To other dear sister-friends: Dale Miller, Jenny Francis, Bea Beasley and Jenn Parkes. Thank you for your love, friendship and help with review, feedback and editing. I deeply appreciate your knowledge, wisdom and understanding.

Cate Jones

Chief Editor's Foreword

I am so grateful that Cate has found the courage and strength to finally tell her story. Because it is not just "her story".

This is a story so much bigger than Cate. She tells it now – not just for her own personal reasons – but also for the sake of all of us who have experienced deep trauma in response to mental, physical, emotional and spiritual abuse, at the hands of those who had promised to love, honor, protect and cherish us…

This is also our story.

Until being asked by Cate to review this book prior to its publication, I had never been able to put words to the traumatic consequences of what I had been through as a young woman – especially the question of "why did I let this happen to me?" Back then, I'd never heard the term "trauma bond" – yet I understood and lived daily with the deeply scarring impacts that unhealthy, abusive relationships have upon our very souls, and how hard they can be to break free from. How long it takes to heal…

In my case I buried the shame I could not name - the trauma and guilt - until it almost buried me! Then my beautiful Savior pulled me up from the all engulfing muck I was bogged and drowning in, and redeemed, healed and restored me.

He showed me Truth and gave me His strength to walk in it. He gave me back my life - He truly set me free.

It was instant, and yet it was a long painful process to learn to walk fully in that freedom. How wonderful it would have been back then to have had a testimony like Cate's – to know I was not alone – that there was a well-lit path already worn between my Egypt and the Promised Land.

This testimony of Cate's is not an easy read. She kept extensive journal notes throughout the years of her difficult sojourn, describing in detail the misery of her daily life under the bondage and slavery of her domestic abuse situation. I have found that many of what were my own patterns of self-destructive behavior are mirrored in her account. Her testimony is an accurate description of the downward spiral which results from the type of abuse she lived through.

And what in some ways may be as bad, or even worse than the abuse Cate has documented, were some of the "treatments" inflicted upon her by the medical system in New Zealand at that time, in their attempts to "fix her" – almost destroying her instead. I am not a clinician, but having worked in the Mental Health system here in Australia, that such a barbaric and inhumane treatment as Electroconvulsive Therapy – "Electroshock Treatment" – is still widely in use even in this day, is truly horrifying. This is nothing other than the intentional infliction of often permanent traumatic brain injury on a human being, to effect a "cure", to make them "normal". I have witnessed the soul destroying after effects, just as Cate's harrowing account describes….

If you are currently walking through such trauma as described in this book – please, keep reading – don't lose hope - keep walking. The dark road described in the first half of this book serves to highlight the wonder of the magnificent and glorious life-giving light at the end of the tunnel.

It has taken Cate fifteen years to come to a place of feeling safe and secure enough to share her story. Her work offers a beacon of light and hope, pointing a way through the darkness, with inspiration and encouragement to grasp hold of the redeeming love of our merciful and loving Creator, Who is calling all of us to walk with Him in the fulness of the blessings of the Promised Land.

It is my prayer for you, dear reader, that as you see yourself in this story – whether as the abused, or the abuser - you too will look to the source of the abundant life you so desperately want and need – The Living Word – Yeshua our Messiah – Yehovah the Son. Allow yourself to dare believe the Truth – you *are loved*, you *are worthy* – He gave His life to rescue, redeem and restore you, too.

Rae Lloyd-Jones, January 2025

Caution:

The description of abuse in this book may be uncomfortable for some Readers.

Introduction

I have set before you life and death, blessing and cursing; therefore choose life!
Deuteronomy 30:19

Do you know that God's Word shows you, and gives you, His divine power to overcome the effects of abuse, trauma, and bondage in your life?

God's Word tells the Bible story of the Exodus - the Israelites' liberation from the **abuse, trauma, and bondage** they experienced in Egypt. The Israelites then met God on **Mount Sinai**. Here, God encouraged them to make a corporate and individual choice to be ***blessed rather than cursed***, so that they and their descendants might ***cross into the Promised Land***. This same choice is ours to make today. It is a choice for all generations.

I chose ***life and blessing,*** and it was this choice - this truth - that has set me free from the effects of abuse, trauma and bondage.

The Promised Land was indeed a physical place which the Israelites were given to put down roots and put up houses. But it was more than that. It was a place of covenant with God to serve Him freely and partake of His blessings. And so it is also *our* place of freedom, purpose, destiny, and… partaking of our Heavenly Father's blessings.

The 'Promised Land' is a framework for an entire society, nation, even world covenant relationship with our Creator. One of *good*, not evil. The 'Promised Land' reveals our personal and loving, covenant relationship with God.

The overarching theme of this book and the one that will follow, is the paradigm shift of coming out of 'Egypt' - the place of abuse, trauma and bondage - and crossing into the 'Promised Land'.

In fact, the Apostle Paul says of the Israelites and the Exodus:

...all these things happened to them as examples,
and they were written for our admonition,
upon whom the ends of the ages have come.
1 Corinthians 10:11

I will therefore tell the story of the Israelite's Exodus and their journey to the Promised Land, as it relates to all of us, through my own personal journey. A very real life-journey that took me to the very real Mount Sinai.

Therefore, this is not simply *my story*, my unraveling and restoration, it is *everyone's story*. Your life may or may not have similarity to mine, but we have all experienced and witnessed abuse, trauma and bondage of some sort - in our own life, in our family, or in the world around us. *Sin,* of course, is most certainly a universal bondage that *God wants to set us all free from!*

Some readers will be experiencing abuse, trauma or bondage even as they begin this book, or, be at the beginning of the healing process. If this is you, please know the light *is* at the end of the tunnel, but it truly is a process that will take time. I pray this book will help awaken and grow God's divine power in you, as you use God's Word to make it happen!

I have written this book so my children might also be set free by knowing the truth (John 8:32) and seeing God's divine power. **I have changed the names of my children and ex-husband. Other individual's names have also been changed, and I have used *'Smith'* as my family name.** So, it will be ***'Smith & Jones'*** throughout this book.

In 2020, I started to learn about the Hebraic roots of my Christian faith. I now prefer to use God's actual name - Yehovah - and our Messiah's Hebrew name - Yeshua Ha'Mashiach (Jesus the Messiah) when reflecting on this story.

*****

I wrote my first book some years ago. The reason for writing it was to exonerate my husband Jack, who had convinced me that he was my 'savior,' and that the cause of my anorexia, depression and suicidality, was not because of him. It was my parents' fault. It took me many years to realize his behavior was sick, as well as emotionally and sexually abusive.

It deeply grieved me to realize I allowed the blame of my illness to be laid on my parents. Many years down the road, after a disastrous marriage with Jack, I sifted the evidence and saw Jack as he really was, and my parents as they really were.

Prior to meeting Jack, I was fully functioning, physically vibrant and mentally well, competent, and strong in my Christian faith. For a number of years, I had lived away from my parents and hometown, successfully finishing my studies to become a Registered Nurse (R.N.). I had then relocated to the South Island of New Zealand to take up my first R.N. position. There, I once more established an independent adult life and integrated into a new faith community.

Then I met Jack…

The domestic abuse target *can be anyone…*
And contrary to the opinions of those who
don't know how abuse works,
she ***isn't targeted because she can't stand***
up for herself or has low self-esteem.
In fact, most abuse targets are not co-dependent at all.
Most of them have been wired from birth with some
powerful personality traits that serve them well*…*
But these same traits, when under the
influence of a toxic person,
are exploited in profound ways in order to
devastate them and render them powerless.
That's right, ***most victims are targeted for their strengths!***
Natalie Hoffman - Is It Me?

Within the year of meeting Jack, we were married. **After two and a half years of marriage** I was diagnosed with Anorexia Nervosa. I had not been anorexic or had any other illness prior to marriage, nor had I taken any psychiatric medications. However, after three years with Jack I was seriously unwell with anorexia, major depression and anxiety. This would lead to six hospitalizations, four suicide attempts and almost twenty years of prescription medication for depression and anxiety.

Jack, the doctors, and therapists all concurred over time that it was due to issues from my childhood. It was difficult enough for my parents to see their daughter suffering like this, but it was made more difficult having the blame for my distress and mental illness laid at their feet. I had become a weak, needy woman, incapable of making decisions, dependent upon Jack.

What got me to this? What got me to hate myself, starve myself, and try to end my life? When I married Jack, I had no clue that anything like this would happen. Was I naive about marriage? Overly naive about life? No, I was 'normal' enough. Jack, it turned out, was not. I tried hard to please Jack. My intention was to love him within the sacred bonds of marriage. Jack's intention was to take complete control of me, my mind and my life. I gave up all my control to Jack.

Eighteen months prior to the end of our twenty-two-year marriage I had gained sufficient insight and spiritual strength, and had figured out what was going on in the relationship. I re-established my personal boundaries and took back my personal power. At this point I made the decision to immediately stop taking all the psychiatric medications I had taken for much of our marriage. I went cold-turkey off the anti-depressants, and the addictive sleeping and anti-anxiety medications. As a result I felt better than I had in a long, long time.

I was back to being a fully functioning, physically strong, mentally well, and competent woman, who had not ever abandoned her faith. However, I was with a husband who had become extremely angry with me for denying him power and control over my life.

The Dog Story

I am keenly aware of how others may have viewed my relationship with Jack. Outwardly, he was a devoted husband who appeared to be very loving and self-sacrificing for me through all my trials with depression, anxiety and anorexia. **Please keep in mind:** I did not have any of those problems before I married Jack, *and* people who viewed our relationship did not know how healthy I used to be, *and* Jack got a lot of power out of telling others how sick I was.

Jack was like a cruel dog owner and sadly, I was the dog…

To everyone else he seems to love his dog, but no one knows he breaks the dog's legs. Instead of taking the dog to have the broken legs set, or simply allowing the dog's legs to heal and get strong again, he does everything he can to maintain the dog's immobility.

But he sure seems to be good to that dog! He keeps the dog covered with a blanket. He lays her beside the fire at night to keep her warm. He brings her food and always makes sure her water bowl is close by and full. The man is so attentive to the dog, that his family and friends look on in awe at just how committed, loyal, and amazing he is to care so well for his dog. The dog is desperate for her master's care. The dog licks her master's hand and believes her broken bones are punishment for something she did not understand.

The dog is now totally dependent upon her master. "What would happen to me," the dog thinks, "if master does not feed me while I cannot move. I would starve. There is no one else who would want me. My master told me so. I am in such pain, and he is so kind and loving to me. I am so grateful for his love and commitment. I am sorry to have to put him through all this trouble. What a bad dog I am. I owe him my life!"

Then one day, the dog decides she wants to get up and walk, maybe even run and play! This angers the master because it will change everything. "How dare she!" He had thought the dog *loved* him! "She was completely safe and cared for with me - now she will run away!" the master seethes.

When the dog finds her way free and realizes that using her legs makes her happy, she *does* try to run away. The master's family and friends look on and exclaim, "What an ungrateful dog! After all he has done for her! How dare the dog do that to him!"

The master is so angry that he now wants to destroy the dog. Everyone feels the no-good dog deserves it, and they feel sorry for her master. What a tragedy for one 'so good' to have to deal with a dog 'so unreasonably difficult.' Because the dog does not want to come near him, he cannot destroy her. He tells his friends, family and neighbors how bad she is so no one will want her.

This is not who the master has become. It is who the master always was.

> *...**when she finally tells the truth** about what's happening to her **friends or Church leaders, she is shot down and punished, adding to the cognitive dissonance that already plagues her.***
> **Natalie Hoffman** - Is It Me?

*****

In reflection, writing the earlier book was me trying to be as honest about my story as I was allowed to be by my husband. It was '*all my parent's fault*.' Mum and Dad had been very good parents, and their love for me never wavered. Ever. In their hurt and pain, they did not retaliate by abandoning me or casting me aside. They did not angrily attempt to talk sense into me. They just kept on loving me and letting me know they would always be there for me. Never did an unloving word pass from their lips to me. All during the emotional and sexual abuse I was caught up in - my parent's love for me never wavered.

My restored relationship with Mum and Dad was the proof that they were not the cause of my illness and distress. If Mum and Dad had been abusers, they would still have been that way. Abusers abuse.

That is what they do. Mum and Dad were loving, kind and concerned, and they continued to love me through it all.

My father passed away on the 22nd of October 2017. He was seventy-eight years old. I love and miss him very much.

The Unbinding of The Book!

I had destroyed all the remaining copies of my earlier book, except for one. This one copy I had placed in a red plastic bag and tightly bound the package with packing tape. I did not *ever* want to see it again or have anyone read it. I had placed it amongst my belongings where it was hidden even from myself - so painful was the memory of that time.

In May of 2022 I finally had the courage to unbind the book, to face the pain, sorrow, shame, guilt and regret that I felt. Until this time, I had bound everything tightly. The memories were more than I could handle. Because of this, I had not ever apologized to Mum and Dad for the blame I had wrongly put upon then. They had eagerly restored their relationship with me - no questions asked and no apology necessary. Now, more than two decades later, with the unbinding of the book, I was distraught at not having apologized.

I called Mum to make amends. On the phone that day, Mum received my apology and received it on Dad's behalf too. She told me that she and Dad had forgiven me long ago, and nothing had been held against me. They knew things were not right or good in my marriage. I marveled at how Mum and Dad had never retaliated or demanded apologies. Just like our Heavenly Father. I was in tears, along with Mum. My emotions about what had happened in those years were unraveling. I was unraveling.

I am writing this book because of that unraveling.

Scripture says:

For we do not wrestle against flesh and blood,
but against principalities, against powers,
against the rulers of the darkness of this age,
against spiritual hosts of wickedness in the Heavenly places.
Ephesians 6:12

This book is not a good-person-verse-bad-person story. Nor is it about mankind simply doing good things or bad things. There is another player at large in this story, indeed all our stories, as there was for the Israelites in Egypt. This is Satan. In Scripture, Satan is also called: The Adversary, The Tempter, The Accuser, Murderer, Father of Lies, Prince of Power of the Air, Béelzebub, and Belial, among others.

When Adam and Eve disobeyed Yehovah in the Garden, they yielded their God-given authority and dominion over all created things on the Earth, to this foul entity called Satan.

Satan brought the curse of sin and death, and Yeshua once-and-for-all broke the curse of sin and death when He was crucified, died and was resurrected. Yeshua reclaimed what Adam and Eve yielded to that cunning snake Satan in the Garden of Eden. **Yeshua reclaimed our spiritual authority and dominion over the Earth and Satan.**

This authority is given back to all who are born-again of the Spirit of Yehovah. It is then, that we are delivered from the power of darkness:

He has delivered us from the
power of darkness and conveyed us into
the kingdom of the Son of His love,
in whom we have redemption through His blood,
the forgiveness of sins.
Colossians 1:13-14

Once we are born-again, we are no longer subject to the power of darkness. In other words, while we are still ***in*** this world, we are no longer ***of it***! Satan and his power of darkness can no longer hold us.

That is critical truth for us. Yet, how many of us know this? I mean, *really* know this? And how many of us live in this understanding with victory over Satan?

Deception is the enemy's deadliest weapon,
but with the power of the Kingdom,
we can rise above it and live a life of abundance and victory.
Dr. Diana Morgan

We can be like the big elephant with innate strength, who still thinks they are a powerless baby elephant tethered to a stake!

When we are living in our reclaimed God-given power, dominion and authority, we can look back on our lives and see what might have been different, or what might never have happened! This surely has been the case for me. Even so, Yehovah promises to ***use all things together for good*** in our lives (see Romans 8:28), and *what Satan means for evil, Yehovah will use for good*, as Joseph stated to his brothers (see Genesis 50:20).

Behind all the people in our lives who have sought to harm us in any way, is Satan. When I married Jack, I was young and not spiritually seasoned. So, while Jack was exercising his agenda that caused great harm to me, Satan had his own diabolical agenda to *steal from me, kill me, and destroy me*, because he did not want me to fulfill my God-given destiny! He did this by exploiting Jack's weaknesses, insecurities, brokenness, wounded-ness, and sin.

Many times, it looked like Satan *had* destroyed me, but he could not because I was in a covenant-relationship with Yehovah through Yeshua, who had promised He would, *never leave me or forsake me* (see Hebrews 13:5). And…Yehovah did keep that promise of *using all things for good in my life!*

Many of us have not known our spiritual authority or used it as we should. The authority that would have allowed us to overcome the Satan and have him under our feet where he belongs. Our victory over the enemy is always certain when we know his tactics, when we stand in faith, when we wear our spiritual armor, and use our spiritual weapons— because *we **are** more than conquerors through Him who loved us and gave Himself for us!* (see Romans 8:31-39)

Whether we are born-again disciples of Yeshua the Messiah or not, Satan is the enemy of all our souls. He and his cohorts are opportunists, always looking to steal, kill and destroy that which is not protected!

The thief Satan comes to steal and kill and destroy;
I, Yeshua, have come that they may have life
and have it to the full.
John 10:10

So there is the human face of an abuser, and a greater enemy Satan with the forces of darkness, who is also at large. When Jack hurt and harmed me, he played right into Satan's hand.

God's abiding Presence, and the Scriptures are the best roadmap available as we live this earthly life. The stories of the Israelite's Sojourn, the Exodus and Sinai, parallel my search - *our search* - for the Promised Land, and are a *"lamp to our feet and a guide to our path."* (Psalm 119:105)

The Word of God has literally rescued me. That is because **the Bible is a supernatural book!** When we read the Scriptures, the words can *fly off the page* at us, because it is **the LIVING WORD of Yehovah**.

For the Word of God is living and powerful,
and sharper than any two-edged sword,
piercing even to the division of soul and spirit,
and of joints and marrow,
*and is **a discerner of the thoughts and intents of the heart**.*
Hebrews 4:12

I would have surely died without the Word of God! It has healed me. It has guided me through challenges and deepest darkest valleys. It has been a vital source of spiritual nourishment. It has provided me with wisdom, insight and direction. It has been a source of comfort and hope in times of overwhelming grief, loss, pain, trouble and despair. The Word of God has reminded me that the One who made me is always with me, that He is Sovereign, and that He has a plan to redeem and restore me, and my children's lives.

The Exodus story is one of *many* Biblical paradigms i.e. blueprints or archetypes, that have relevance for my life and yours today. In our personal journeys, as well as in our nations, the experiences of either the Israelites or the Egyptians are being played out. We can see this in our *struggles and successes* or in our ultimate *demise*.

There is nothing new under the sun! Satan took full advantage of the situation that played out between Jack and me. He used Jack's inclination and desires to control and abuse, and mine to submit and surrender my power, to get us on a treacherous downward path. Satan will do that to you too if you are not prepared. This book is to encourage you and help you prepare.

In the telling of my story, I will hold up the Biblical passages of the Exodus, and the journey to the Promised Land, as instruction and inspiration. I have done this because the Exodus story is the paradigm of what we all must go through, and the reason for it. Feast or famine is ours to choose. As Moses said to the Israelites when they were camped on the plains of Moab, opposite Jericho, on the other side of the Jordan, we must choose between *blessing and cursing*. Between *life and death*. Beloved, **choose life!** (see Deuteronomy 30:19).

*****

The Promise

After these things the word of Yehovah came to Abram in a vision,
saying, "Do not be afraid, Abram. I AM your shield,
your exceedingly great reward."

On the same day Yehovah made a covenant with Abram, saying:
"To your descendants I have given this land,
from the river of Egypt to the great river, the River Euphrates."
Genesis 15:1,18

CHAPTER 1

In The Beginning: Dawn Of The World

In the beginning *God created the Heavens and the Earth.*
Genesis 1:1

Gisborne is the most easterly city on our planet, so those who live there are blessed with the first glimpse of our rising sun each day. Gisborne is on the East Cape of New Zealand's North Island. So, when the rising sun hits Gisborne… BOOM! A brand-new day in the world has dawned! This is where I grew up, and it was a great place to come into the world.

Water, Water, Water!

I grew up in a small island nation, in a town on the coast, in a house by the beach, with a pool in the back yard! Almost every day in summer I swam at the beach, or was in the pool at home, school, or swim club. If not, I was probably in the boat with Dad. Water, water, water. It was such a huge part of my life.

For many of my adult years I swam laps for fitness three or four times a week. I also sat poolside as my children had their swim lessons from preschool age until they became accomplished swimmers. My most fun memories in the water as an adult were with my children, as well as white water rafting in New Zealand, and kayaking adventures in New Zealand and Australia. The happiest times in life have been in the water. Still to this day, just put me in water and I am happy!

Pharaoh's daughter named him Moses [Pulled Out] and said,
"I pulled him out of the water."
Exodus 2:10

There were other times in my adult life, however, when I was truly *un*happy in *the water*. I felt emotionally and spiritually that I was in deep, tumultuous water when I went through two years of Family Court proceedings, for example, and experienced extreme parental alienation from my children. Even so, the physical water was the one place that helped sooth my anguished soul. I would swim way out into the ocean, past the breaking waves, and there - float on my back as the waves rolled gently under my body. It seemed quite possible that I raised the level of the ocean by crying bucket loads of tears. It was being in the water away from the land that gave me some respite from all that was hurting me so badly. Even into the winter months when the water was freezing cold, I would put on my wetsuit and escape to the water. And later… Yehovah miraculously *parted the deep waters* for my ***Red Sea Road.***

"He drew me out of deep waters" (Psalm 18:16, NIV) describes a powerful experience of deliverance and rescue. This phrase is repeated in various forms throughout the Psalms, emphasizing the magnitude of Yehovah's intervention.

Yehovah had saved baby Moses out of the water, and Yehovah saved me out of my *tumultuous waters*! Moses had a destiny to fulfill, and *so did I!* I was yet to discover that much of my life would follow the challenges of Moses and the Israelites during the Exodus.

But let's start from the beginning.

*****

A Love Story

My father finished his building apprenticeship when he was 18, and he was anticipating going to the World Scout Jubilee Jamboree in England. He was diagnosed with a serious heart defect, however, and heart surgery was necessary to save him from an early death. The heart specialist told him, *"If you want to travel the world, Young Man, you had better do it now."* So, Dad decided to travel before having surgery, and he boarded a ship sailing from New Zealand to Europe for a two-year stint of work and holiday. It began with the Jamboree he attended with some 50,000 Scouts from 82 nations. Dad was a

Queen Scout, which was the highest youth award achievable in the Scouting movement in the Commonwealth realms. So, being at the jamboree was, for him, a dream come true. The year was 1957.

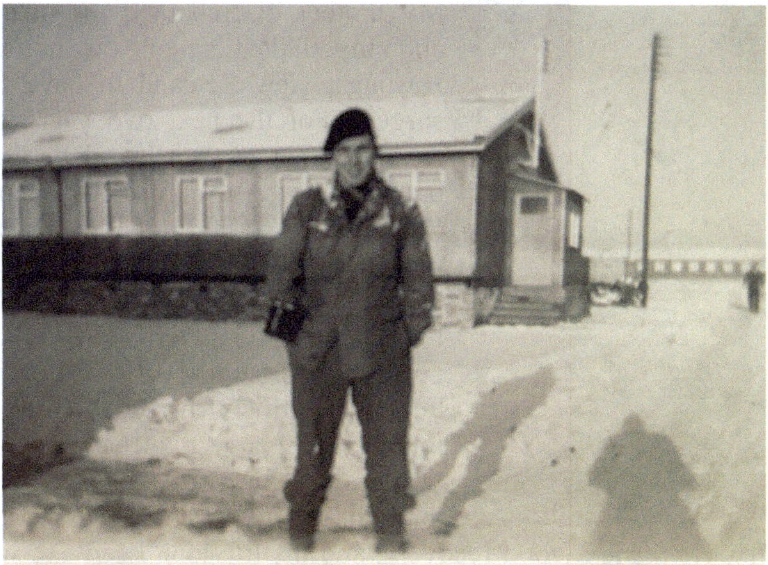

Dad at the World Scout Jubilee Jamboree, England 1957

It was not difficult for Dad to find employment as a builder as he traveled Europe. Furthermore, when in Germany and commuting on the train to the worksite each day, he used the time to teach himself to speak the language. He always had a lot of fun with language and could convincingly mimic accents and people's speech quirks. Consequently, even though he learned from a book, he spoke the German language with such finesse that German folk thought he was from a particular part of Germany!

Returning home on a ship from England to New Zealand, Dad met and fell in love with my mother, *"a young English beauty,"* as Dad described her - after he tripped over her feet when she was sunbathing on the promenade deck! Mum was a beautiful, brave young woman who had just graduated as a Registered Nurse (R.N.) and midwife. She had accepted an offer from the Australian Government to have free passage to Australia in exchange for working two years as a nurse in the Australian Outback. To this day, I am surprised and inspired

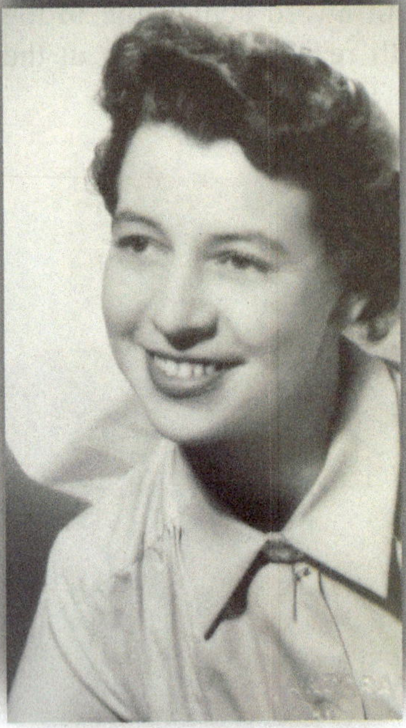

that inside my quiet and reserved Mum, was a brave and adventurous spirit.

My mother disembarked in Australia, and my father sailed on home to Hastings, New Zealand to have heart surgery. For the next two years, their romance grew as their love letters went back and forth across the Pacific Ocean. A beautiful black and white photo of my Mum as a nursing graduate sat on Dad's hospital bedside locker in a small silver frame (which is now in my home). Dad's love-smitten heart for this English beauty he intended to marry may have been the thing that kept his heart beating through the risky and invasive heart surgery. He made a good recovery, and his life-long keepsake was a dramatic crescent-shaped scar extending from the top of his back to his lower ribs on his left side.

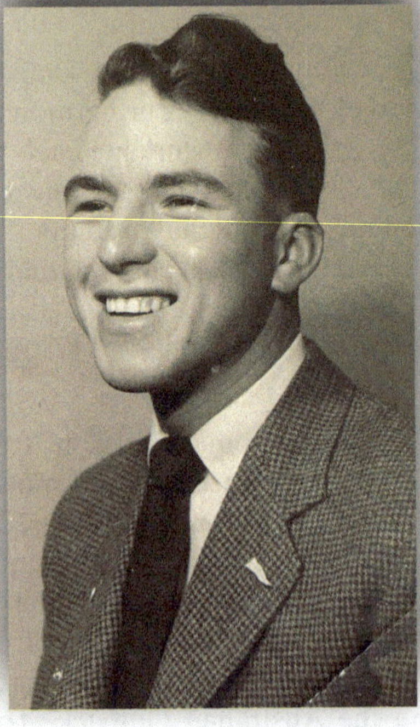

Prior to marriage, Dad bought his grandparents' house located on a large piece of land by the beach in Gisborne. He reconfigured it into three separate flats (apartments). One was to be where he and Mum would live, and the other two would be rentals. Then, in 1960 when my mother's two-year-contract ended, Dad boarded a ship bound for Australia where he and Mum were reunited. Together, they boarded another ship headed to England for their wedding - where they would become Mr. and Mrs. 'Smith'!

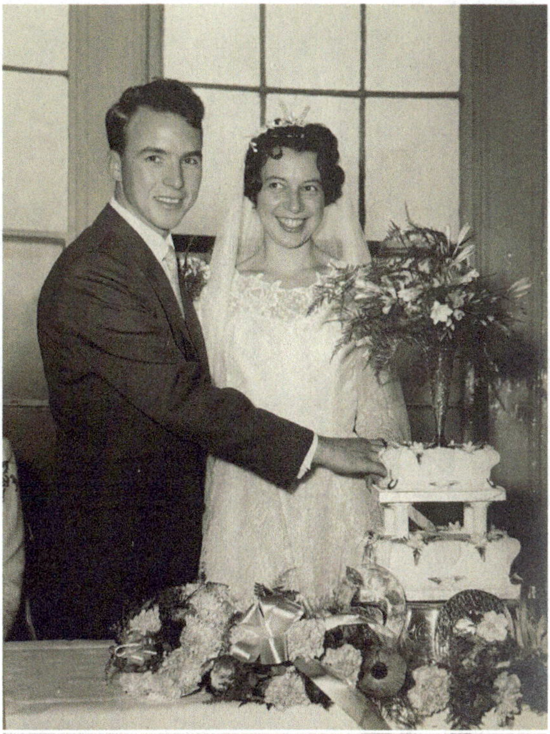

Mum & Dad. Married in Leeds, Yorkshire, England, 1960

I love to tell their story! Its marvelously romantic how a charming, young Kiwi bloke on his voyage home from a major life adventure across the globe met a demure young English nurse who happened to be on the same ship and on her way to the Australian Outback. Their courtship consisted of two years of sending letters back and forth between New Zealand and Australia, and then they were married. It's amazing!

I am ever imagining what these years must have been like for Mum. She left her homeland…sailed six weeks on board a ship as a young single woman…met a handsome young man who swept her off her feet…on her way to a vastly different land on the other side of the world…where she experienced an unknown culture, climate, people and language - among the Aboriginal people - as she started her professional life as a new nurse midwife…faced the great tragedy of losing her Outback nursing friend to suicide…returned to England to

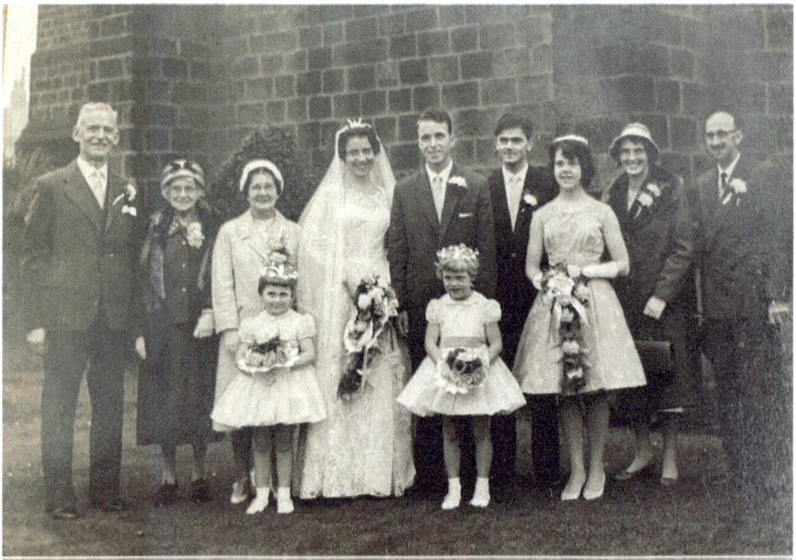

**Mum's parents and grandmother on the left.
Dad's parents on the right. Dad's parents mortgaged their home in New Zealand to sail to England and attend the wedding.**

marry…enjoyed a six-week honeymoon on board a ship once again… arrived in New Zealand…in the early weeks of pregnancy…and had to reorient, adjust and navigate another whole new country, culture, climate, people and family. How incredible! Mum is now 91 years old, and in a recent conversation, I told her how brave and adventurous, loving and hardworking she has been in her life. She laughed and said she could hardly believe that she did all the things she had done, especially in the first years of leaving her parents and homeland of England.

My mother is still living an amazing life. She is no longer raising her six children, or knitting all our winter jerseys, or making the best homemade bread ever, or filling kitchen cupboards with canned fruits, beets, chutney, jams, pickles, spaghetti sauce and ginger beer, or writing all the letters she once did. In spite of every limitation she now experiences, however, she continues to live with grace, contentment, and a heart of gratitude. She readily smiles, laughs and expresses thankfulness to God in every conversation that I am still so blessed to have with her.

New Family, New Home

My eldest brother Timothy (Tim) was a honeymoon baby. My second brother Simon came twelve months later. Then I arrived eighteen months after Simon in 1964. Dad had his own building business and Mum juggled caring for three young children with evening midwifery shifts at The Salvation Army Maternity Hospital for unwed mothers. It was there that she delivered a baby girl whose teenage mother asked Mum to adopt her baby. My parents agreed, and they named her Francis (Fran). Mum and Dad were then parents to four children under five years old! All four of us were dedicated to God when we were infants by my parents who exercised their will and determination to bring us up in the ways of God.

We lived in a two-bedroom flat (apartment) by the beach until I was five years old. The second bedroom was small and narrow. It could only fit two sets of bunk beds placed end to end for us four children. There was a small window in the room that I could open and look out of from my top bunk bed. When I was put to bed at night, I would watch Dad from that small window as he built our big, brand-new house on the back of the property. Dad worked hard on the house, using every daylight hour until the sun set.

One particular hot summer night, I was watching the sun through the open window as it set behind Dad while he worked. Mesmerized by the sun, I fell asleep. Not only did I fall asleep, I also fell out the window! Not only did I fall out the window, but I remained asleep! Dad, not one for being unduly concerned about things, found me and calmly assessed that I was *just a sleeping four-year-old child on the ground at night who had fallen out of her bedroom window.* He simply lifted me up and put me back through the open window into my bed. I had remained sound asleep with no injury or harm done! Then the sun rose the next morning to start the world off again! The house was soon finished, and we moved into our big brand-new, four-bedroom split level house. Dad would later add two more bedrooms when our family grew further.

Family Faith

Christian faith was central to everything in our family. My father's family was as committed and active as any family could be in the evangelical church of The Salvation Army. And our family was no different. In fact, I was the fourth generation to belong to The Salvation Army. Dad was a solid Christian who lived out his faith every single day. It was, therefore, a tremendous joy to him, in their first year of marriage, the day Mum also chose to follow Jesus Christ and have a personal relationship with Him. Mum then joined Dad in the ranks of The Salvation Army, and proudly donned her own Salvation Army uniform.

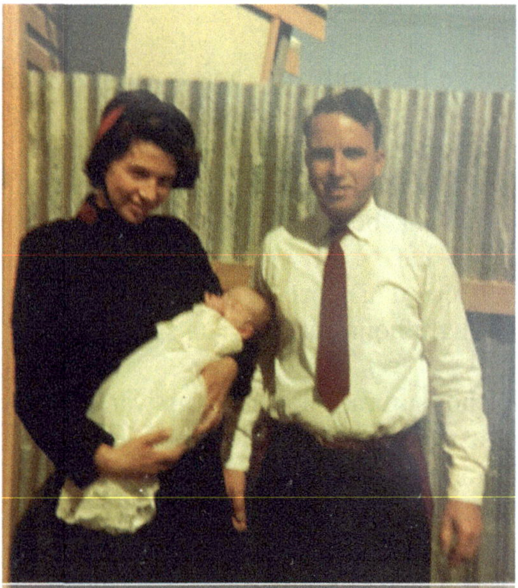

Mum and Dad with me the day I was dedicated to Yehovah. My parents wearing their Salvation Army uniforms.

I was eight years old when I made that most important life decision to follow Jesus Christ. My understanding was simple and genuine - I believed that Jesus loved me and died on a cross so that I could be forgiven for the wrong things I had done. In that moment I was born-again by the Spirit of Yehovah. I was adopted into the family-line and blessings of Abraham. This began a faith journey with my Creator and Savior—a journey that I am still on more than five decades later.

As a child, I was yet unaware of what this would mean for my life, and how the Promised Land of Canaan would relate to me!

"I will make my promise to you
and your descendants
for generations to come as an
everlasting promise.
I will be your God and the God of
your descendants.
I am also giving this land where
you are living—
all of Canaan—to you and your
descendants
as your permanent possession.
And I will be your God."
Genesis 17:7-8

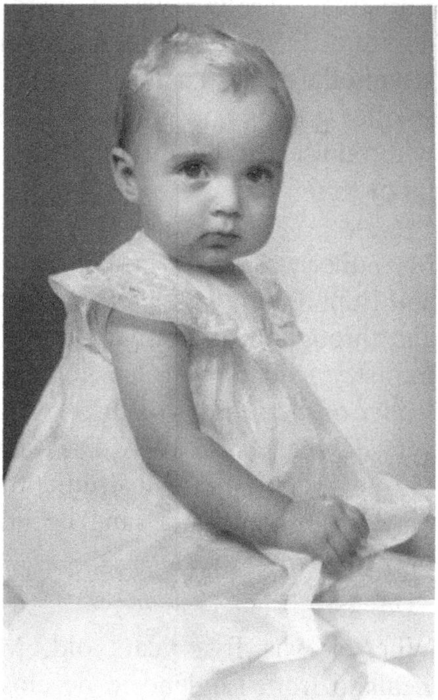

The Salvation Army Corps Church life did a lot to shape me since it was central to our family's life. As children, we attended Sunday School each Sunday morning, as well as both the morning and evening worship services. There were two evangelical "open air'" meetings on Sundays led by the Corps brass band where the gospel message was shared in music, Scripture and impromptu salvation testimonies. There was also an open-air meeting in the town's main street every Friday night when the gospel message was shared with late night shoppers. Throughout the week, there were rehearsals for junior and senior band, junior and senior singing groups, tambourine practice, youth group activities, and Corps Cadets - a teenage discipleship program.

My family prayed together. In addition to praying before our meals, we prayed together before leaving for school each morning. Mum would gather us children in the kitchen, where we stood in a circle and prayed for things such as school tests and exams, bike tires not getting punctured, things we were thankful for, etc. Before being “dismissed” by Mum, one of us would get to take a promise out of the Bible promise box and read it out.

Christmas caroling was a major event each year. Throughout the month of December, the band would go out caroling every weeknight around the town. Then on Sunday mornings, the band would split into smaller groups and go far and wide to share the Christmas message with families and communities in the surrounding rural areas. It was a lot of fun!

My father was a very gifted musician - both vocally and on the Cornet and Euphonium (brass valved instruments). From the time I was little and throughout the remainder of his life, Dad held significant music ministry leadership roles in the Corps. For many years he was the leader of the senior vocalists. And then, for many more years until the very day he passed away, Dad was the brass Band Master. My mother did not play a brass instrument like the rest of our family, but she played the piano and sang beautifully. My siblings and I learned to play the piano, too.

When I was five years old, Mum’s parents immigrated to New Zealand from England to be close to their only child. They lived in one of the flats next door to us.

When I was ten years old, my parents were asked to foster two little girls. Janie was five years old with special needs, and her sister Jessie was eighteen months old. They were in bad shape from extreme neglect, and needed a permanent, loving home. Our family grew to eight, keeping my mother busy with six children. She also worked two nursing night shifts on the weekend. While Mum caught sleep during the daytime on weekends, I would look after Janie and Jessie. I felt very motherly towards Jessie as she and I were particularly close for the first seven years of her life.

When I was thirteen years old, Dad’s parents - Grandma and Grandpa 'Smith' - retired from their grocery store business in Christchurch, New Zealand. Then they came to live in Gisborne as well. So, we had all four of our grandparents in Gisborne! I was especially close to my paternal grandparents, and it was Grandma 'Smith' who primarily taught me to sew with the sewing machine. During some of my high school years I would regularly stay Thursday nights with Grandma and Grandpa 'Smith' just to have special time with them.

Believe it or not, there was rhyme and rhythm in all the comings and goings of our rambunctious household. My siblings and I walked or rode our bikes to school each day. We did our homework and our chores. We all played team sports and were in swim club. We had daily piano lessons and practices along with singing and band practices. We all followed Dad's lead into the Baden-Powell movement and became cubs, boy scouts, brownies, and girl guides. Dad was a scout leader for the years that my brothers were in the scouts. Our home and meal table were open to strangers, extended family and school friends. We had plenty of family holidays or day trips where we would camp, swim, boat, and fish. And, because Dad's side of the family lived in other parts of New Zealand, we also spent some holidays visiting them or having them visit us. Camping with our extended family was a lot of fun. Our family dog, whichever it was at the time, was mixed in amongst our family activities as well.

Bike cleaning with Jessie

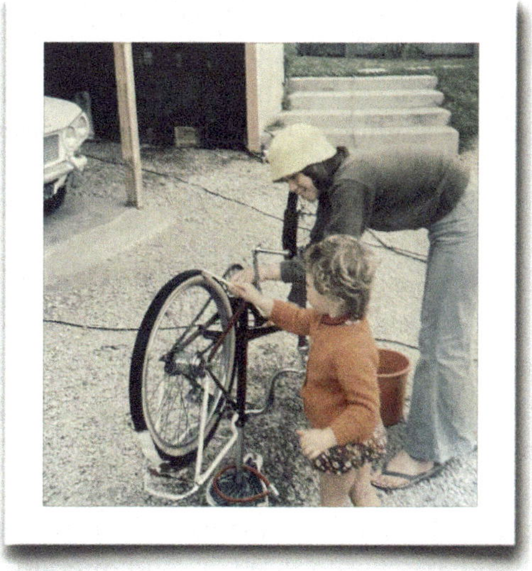

A couple of memories of Dad...

Dad was a Registered Master Builder, and it seemed to me that he knew how to fix or solve most anything. He was also a master at soothing irritations and enlivening the atmosphere because of his great heart and spirit. He was funny, and always ready to laugh and see the bright side of things. His wit, impersonations, jokes and laughter were one of the things that characterized him, and this built many bridges into other people's lives.

I remember the time he went to a bank to cash a check, and the bank teller asked him for identification. Without hesitation, Dad pulled out a small mirror from his pocket, looked in it, and said to the teller with a grin, *"Yes, that's me!"*

There was another time when we went on holiday to the Bay of Islands in New Zealand with our tent and boat. We arrived at a destination late in the day, to find that the local camping ground was full. So, we drove a bit further to a pristine beach that had a sign 'NO OVERNIGHT CAMPING.' Dad saw no reason why an unoccupied beach could not be a perfect place for us to stay the night, so we pitched our tent over the sign, and slung our wet beach towels over it! When we had all settled in for the night, a policeman came by with his flashlight and said, we should not be camping there as it was a no overnight camping beach. Dad stepped out of the tent, looked around and said, *"I can't see any 'No Overnight Camping' sign here."* The policeman scratched his head saying, *"I could have sworn there was a sign here somewhere."* With a shrug of his shoulders, the policeman turned and left saying, *"Just be gone by morning."* We had a lot of laughter over that one.

Getting to Work

My parents taught us to work hard and appreciate success. We learned to be resourceful, resilient, and independent. From a young age, my siblings and I all found ways to earn money. Just as soon as we were old enough, we put advertisement flyers in people's letter boxes. Tim and Simon collected and resold soft drink bottles from around the neighborhood and carted them around on a go-cart Dad had made. My brothers also mowed lawns and cleaned old bricks for resale. Simon also stripped and rebuilt old, abandoned bicycles and restored broken washing machines to sell.

My first paid job was as an eight-year-old. Every Saturday I would bake a cake, a batch of biscuits (cookies), and a tray of brownies or some other sweet treat, and Mum would pay me fifteen cents. This started when I received birthday presents of my own baking bowls, a wooden spoon, a sift, measuring cups and spoons, and cookie cutters. Mum even gave me my very own kitchen cupboard to store all my new things! It was a proud day for me. I began to bake eagerly and regularly.

Before I learned to sew on Grandma 'Smith''s treadle machine in middle school, Mum taught me to knit and hand sew when I was six years old. As soon as I had mastered the sewing machine, I enthusiastically took on the responsibility of tending to the family's constant pile of clothes that needed mending. This started my love of sewing and the desire to restore things (anything) that would otherwise be discarded. It was not long before I was making clothes for the family, as well as children's clothes and household items that Mum would sell to her nursing colleagues when she worked her night shifts. I babysat, and I worked Saturday afternoons at a corner store. During school holidays I worked at a toy store, and then later at a restaurant. As my parents had taught us all to tithe, I was proud to take a tenth of everything I earned and put it in the offering plate each Sunday. They also taught us how to set goals and reach them. I earned money for things I wanted or needed, like a new bike, a stereo, bedroom furniture, and an awesome brand-new sewing machine.

During high school I paid off that Bernina sewing machine by taking in sewing repair work and making clothes that I then sold. I spent every possible minute in the sewing nook of my new bedroom that Dad had added to our house. I made countless t-shirts, sweaters, knickers and petticoats. I became a frequent shopper at the Bernina store to replenish my sewing supplies - to the point that the owners asked if I would work for them when I finished school! I decided that was a good thing to do for one year.

I did not do all my work for pay, though. In my high school years, I grew hundreds of different African violet plants of different varieties from single leaves. My small bedroom was full of dozens of potted African Violets in all stages of growth. I would examine them every day to check their growth and was excited with every first leaf that emerged from the soil and every first bud that opened to reveal the color. I did not sell my plants; I gave them to people just to see them smile. That made me smile, too.

Modeling Love

As is plain to see, I had an extremely blessed childhood. And I had good mental and physical health because of that. My parents modeled a loving and caring marriage for us. They worked hard and taught us to do the same. We always had everything we needed, and more besides. Our family was the first family I knew of to get a color television! And when I was thirteen, Mum and Dad took us four older children on a camper van holiday around Australia. I was the first of all my friends to "go overseas!"

Mum and Dad taught me by their example how to show my love for God by loving and caring for others - even if it was costly or inconvenient. I saw how Dad was quick to give practical help to others, both in small ways and in significant ways, like when natural disasters occurred. I remember one time when he took weeks off from work to go to the pacific island nation of Fiji to help them rebuild after it was devastated by a cyclone. I watched him many times as he naturally shared the gospel with others; telling of his faith and trust in a loving Heavenly Father who desired for them to know His love too.

I saw Mum doing things like putting coins in parking meters that had expired just before a Meter Maid issued a parking ticket, taking food to people, sending bereavement cards to people she did not even know but who had lost loved ones, and regularly writing letters of support and encouragement to missionaries around the world. And, of course, I saw my parents bring needy children into our family to love.

Everything my parents did was an extension of their love and loyalty to each other. There were irritations here and there between them, but I cannot recall any arguing or fighting between them. I do not ever remember Dad even being angry with Mum. There was nothing in Dad's nature that was mean or hurtful, so I knew no other way of a husband relating towards his wife. Mum and Dad worked and lived as a team, and valued each other's roles in the relationship. I have loads of memories of Dad kissing and cuddling Mum, of him serenading her, and him bragging about her to anyone who would listen. My Dad was also a writer and a poet. He wrote two books of love poems to my mother! As the years went on, I truly saw how Mum and Dad faced the hard things in their life courageously, honorably, and holding to the faith they professed together.

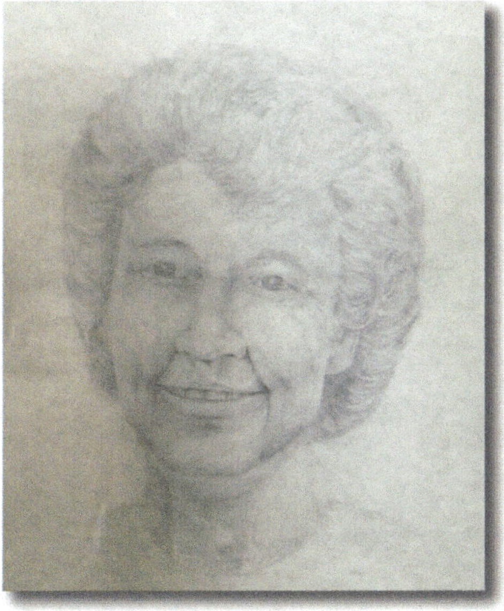

Dad's sketch of Mum

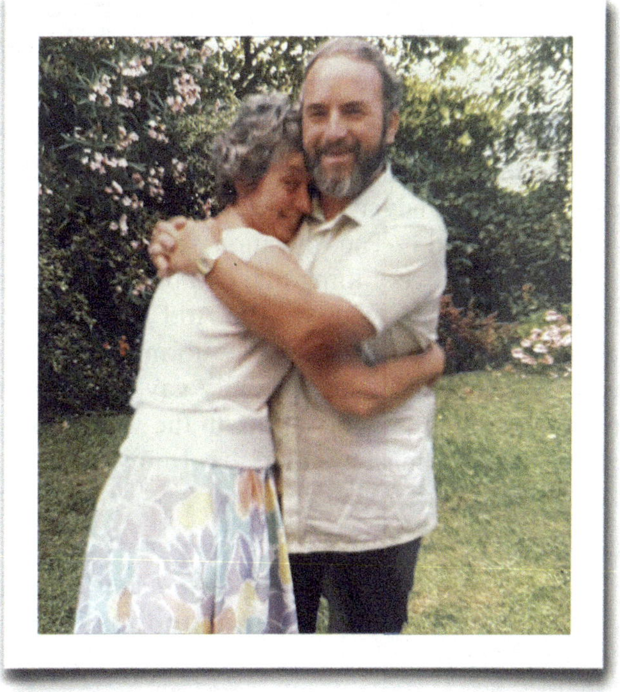

Mum and Dad

*****

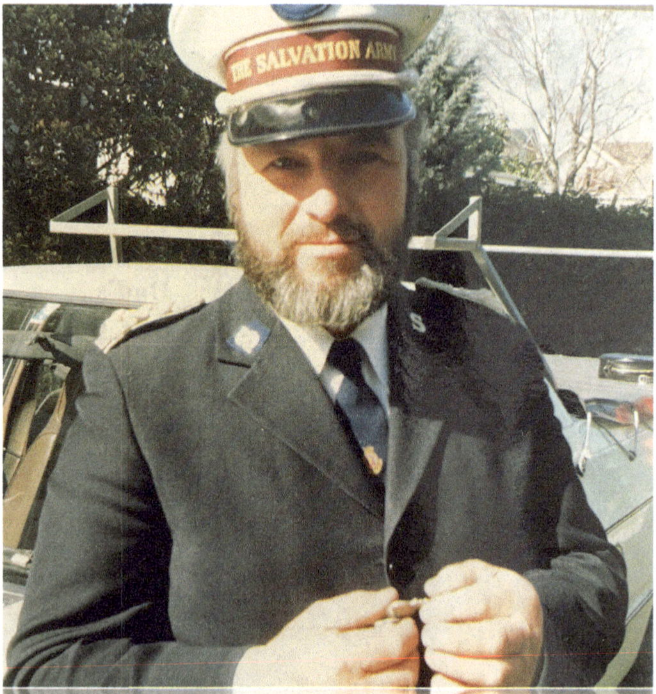

Dad in his Salvation Army Bandmaster's uniform

2024 Flashback: On the 31st of October in 2017, Mum and Dad were together in Sunday morning worship when Dad suffered a massive heart attack and never regained consciousness. He was *"promoted to glory,"* as is said in The Salvation Army, in the very place he loved so much, doing the very thing that had brought endless joy, meaning and purpose to his life. Dad was 78. And he was, of course, wearing his Salvation Army bandmaster's uniform. It was 56 years after Dad's heart surgery that his heart finally gave out. At that moment, he got promoted to being a worshipper in the very presence of his Heavenly Father! His bandmaster's cap, that I now have, is a precious treasure of my loving Dad.

I dedicate this book, *Red Sea Road to Sinai,* to Mum and Dad

*****

At the end of 1981 I graduated high school. And so I entered adulthood, having had a full, healthy and successful childhood.

For the best part of a year, I demonstrated and sold Bernina sewing machines and helped customers with their fabric and haberdashery needs. I also regularly took home sewing repair work for customers which gave me extra income. This enabled me to earn the initial funds I needed to begin nursing school the following year, and to trade up my sewing machine for another new one that was the top of the line. In addition, I had money enough to go to the Pacific Island nation of Tonga to volunteer for three months before my nursing training commenced.

It was not through The Salvation Army or any mission group that I went to the Kingdom of Tonga, and my decision to go to was rather spontaneous. It had come about through a conversation I had with a friend who told me of a Tongan kindergarten teacher, named Hulita, who could use my help in her two village kindergartens. I prayed about it. The Holy Spirit led me to say, *"I'll go!"*

Making this trip on my own at eighteen years old was an exciting way to stretch my wings. Mum and Dad supported my plans, giving every encouragement. I filled two big suitcases with teaching resources, and the New Zealand Public Health Service was willing to give me boxes of high protein dried milk biscuits to take for the kindergarten children.

It was not difficult to live on a beautiful tropical island for three months with easy-going and open-hearted Tongans. I lived in a Tongan village with the kindergarten teacher's extended family. The home was small and simple, and surrounded by coconut palm trees that gave shade and shelter to the outdoor cooking and washing area. Inside the home were three small sleeping areas where we all slept on Tongan woven flax mats. In the living area there were large and more elaborate finely woven decorative mats.

During the week we ate tropical fruit, root vegetables and vermicelli, but on Sunday we ate like kings! Early each Sunday morning the women prepared food for the *umu* (an Earth oven that is a pit in the ground). The men prepared the *umu* and sometimes a spit-roasted piglet too. Once the food was wrapped and safely placed in the coals and hot rocks of the *umu*, it was then covered over with earth. We would then put on our best Tongan clothes and walk to church. Returning two or three hours later, the food would be perfectly baked. In preparation to eat, fresh banana leaves would be laid down like a tablecloth on the floor in our home, and the food set out on top. After prayers of thanksgiving, we partook of the bounty, as we sat cross-legged either side of the food. There was fish, taro, green bananas and other vegetables cooked in coconut cream, and pork or chicken. I've never eaten anything more delicious in my life!

Helping Hulita in the kindergartens was a joy for me. I dearly loved the children and gained far more than I could give in so many ways. I sang in the church choir each Sunday and rehearsed with them mid-week, but as it was all in Tongan, I had no idea what I was singing about other than to know I was praising Yehovah! I'd known only a few Tongan words and phrases when I arrived but was happy to be fully immersed in the Tongan language. Smiles, gestures, laughter and love did a lot to help communication. I joined in and said *"yes"* to every opportunity to share family, village and church life, but said *"no"* to two marriage proposals by Tongan men. It was a truly blessed time. I grew in my faith, and it was there I was baptized. My sojourn in Tonga was an idyllic journey in my life.

My suitcases that were emptied of the things I took for the kindergartens, came back to New Zealand packed full of beautiful handmade gifts from those I said *"goodbye"* to - precious painted tapa clothes, shell necklaces, elaborately embroidered pillowcases and table runners, woven mats and baskets. I was truly blessed. Mum and Dad drove to Auckland to pick me up from the airport when I flew back into the country. I have precious memories and photos of their joy in seeing me again. I felt vibrantly healthy and alive!

As my siblings and I grew up and moved out of our home, we all had our plans and directions. My eldest brother Tim learned the building trade from Dad. He moved away from Gisborne to be closer to his girlfriend. My brother Simon took on the electrical trade and gained his flying credentials - pursuing all sorts of interests and travel. I went off to the Hawkes Bay of New Zealand to become a Registered Nurse (R.N.). Two of my sisters - Fran and Jessie, became teachers.

*****

The Hawkes Bay is most famously known for the devastating 1931 Earthquake that killed 256 people and injured thousands. Dad's parents were among the survivors. Even now, this event remains New Zealand's deadliest natural disaster.

The twin cities of Napier and Hastings were rebuilt. Hastings is where my father grew up, and Napier is the Art Deco capital of world. With a population of 176,000, the Hawkes Bay has beautiful landscapes, a lovely climate, orchards and fine wineries. It was there that I lived for the three years I trained as a nurse.

In this time, I was an active uniformed solider in The Salvation Army Hastings Corps where my father had grown up. I played a tenor horn in the band, sang in the songsters and was the leader of the senior timbrel group. While there were no longer any of my extended family members living in Hastings, it was nice seeing Grandma and Grandpa 'Smith', my father, and my aunts and uncles in the old band photos that hung on the band room wall.

Being a student nurse required a lot of work and study which was challenging for me. However, I really excelled on the wards and in other practical experience with patient care. I guess it was in my blood! Pediatric nursing and community care were my favorite areas, and in my vacation times I was a nurse aid at a maternity hospital. A most marvelous experience was Christmas Day 1984, when as a first -year student nurse, I witnessed the birth of a baby! At this point in my nursing training, I had not yet done any obstetrics.

In my final year, I spent three months as a student nurse in the pediatric ward of Rotorua Hospital. I lived in the nurse's home and was fully involved the Rotorua Salvation Army Corps, an experience I thoroughly enjoyed.

After all the hours of studying for my nursing state final exams, it was a relief to have them behind me and to graduate as a Registered Nurse in general, mental health and obstetric care. I remember the day I held the envelope in my hands, that would tell me whether I had passed or failed my exams. I opened it with fear and trembling. Seeing the word 'PASS' in big bold letters was joy beyond joy!

As well as nursing graduation, I graduated from riding a little yellow scooter to driving a sporty turquoise Datsun hatchback. This, I loaded all my belongings into and drove down to Wellington, crossed over the Cook Strait on a ferry, and continued my journey down the coastline of New Zealand's South Island. My two-day journey ended in Christchurch, the largest city on the east coast of the South Island with a population of 380,000 people.

Never will I forget my first day at Burwood Spinal Injury Hospital wearing my white uniform, white stockings, white shoes, little white cap, red cape and my shiny new R.N. badge. Christchurch was, and still is, a very traditional 'English' city. Consequently, it was the last place in New Zealand to move away from the old-style nurses uniforms. I felt like my mother… as if I was an English nurse! I was no longer just wearing the nurse dress-up costume I had as a child!

I met Jack in the first weeks of being in Christchurch at a planning meeting for leaders of an upcoming Easter camp for Salvation Army youth. While I did not know anyone, most people seemed to know Jack. He was jokingly referred to as 'Mr. Clipboard.' He had this reputation for masterfully conducting youth events through the power of his clipboard! Jack introduced himself to me and appeared to be 'interested' in me. So much so, that his attention was duly noted by others. I was flattered, but my first impression was… he seems a bit arrogant. I chastised myself for making such a quick judgement of him. At Easter camp we had more opportunities to chat, and then… we were dating.

I was a complete novice at dating. While I had previously had the strange and awkward experiences of three men asking me to marry them - two in Tonga and the other at the Hastings Salvation Army Corps, I had not dated them. But in four months Jack and I would become engaged and married five months after that. I was twenty-three when we married.

She is trustworthy, open, honest, and forthright.
She vulnerably shares her inner world with him
in the hope of building a deep, intimate connection...
Natalie Hoffman - Is It Me?

Jack was quick off the mark, and love bombed me! In that first week of dating I received two dozen red roses, delivered to the nurse's station on the ward where I was working. The nursing staff were set abuzz with wanting to know who my admirer was! Though somewhat embarrassed, I was once again flattered. Jack did not hold back from making his intentions known, and this wasn't to be the only bouquet of flowers delivered to me at the hospital. These floral deliveries impressed those I worked with, who wished they had such romantic attention. When Jack introduced me to his parents, I was warmly welcomed into their home— where Jack still lived. The relationship all started so nicely!

It was soon after meeting Jack that he left his bank job to be a Regional Youth Worker for The Salvation Army. This got a tick from me as it lined up with the values I had. In my late teens, I had a spiritual growth spurt and as a result of the work of the Holy Spirit in my life, I had felt a stirring in me towards church or mission work. I was willing and intended to keep my heart open to this. Jack spoke to me of his plans to go to The Salvation Army Training College to become a Salvation Army officer (minister). So, I pondered this possibility in my heart.

2024 Looking Back:
On several occasions in and around that time, I heard Jack tell people, *"I wanted to become a Salvation Army officer, but the problem was I wasn't saved. So, I got saved!"* I remember how this had made people laugh. It was remarkable that at the end of our marriage Jack appeared to have fallen away from his appearance of faith.

More remarkable - shocking even - would be that I would have no experience of Jack and I ever praying together throughout the entirety of our twenty two-year marriage and fifteen years as Salvation Army officers, other than to say grace before a family meal! I have no experience or knowledge of Jack ever praying with me or for me in all my years of sickness and distress, or for our children, or for our greater family, or for others.

We never see these things at the time.

*****

Though I had been well trained as an R.N., starting out as a newbie was very stressful. I remember feeling that I was not managing expectations well. It did not help that there was a significant staff shortage. It meant that as new R.N.s, we were less supported. We even found ourselves being the most senior staff members on a ward, being responsible for the Enrolled Nurses (E.N.s) on our shifts, who had less training than R.N.s. I had more than a few times of being anxious before a shift. I feared the responsibility on my shoulders would be more than I could manage. Ultimately, this led me to find employment as a general practice nurse which I greatly enjoyed.

When Jack was not working and I was not working, we were together. Other than my work time, my one point of separation from Jack was Sunday when I went to church. Since my aunt and uncle were living in Christchurch, I had decided to go to The Salvation Army Corps they attended, which was a different Corps to the one Jack's family attended. Here I established new and separate relationships, played in the band and sang with the songsters. Other than this, my life was quickly melding with Jack's life.

It was somewhat amusing to me to see how different Jack was to my father. Dad was 'organic' in his ways, whereas Jack was 'highly processed' i.e. Jack micro-managed everything. He was forward-planned, backwards-planned and sideways-planned! It meant that if Jack planned to meet me at a certain time, he was there. This was amazing! Dad might have been fifteen or twenty or even thirty minutes late. If Jack had planned a surprise for me, every detail was wonderfully worked out. Dad? Ah…no. If Jack and I were making a trip somewhere, his car had the tires checked, gas tank filled, and insurance all up to date. Dad? Maybe not. If we were going to the beach, Jack would have sunblock, sunhat, umbrella, raincoat, gumboots and snow boots! *(slight exaggeration)* Dad might have swimwear and maybe a towel. In short, Jack strived to control everything around him.

Jack would tell me, *"I need to plan to be spontaneous."* I used to think this was funny, until it wasn't. He was planned and thorough, right down to the last detail. I experienced Mr. Clipboard's super organization and attention to detail as good and positive at first, as it gave me a sense of confidence and security in my new environment.

2024 Looking Back:
Yehovah made me to be a good follower of a good leader. While I would lead if no one else would, I was naturally a follower - a good and loyal one. What I believed was that Jack, the man that I loved, was a 'good' leader. After all, Jack, like my father, was in The Salvation Army. He was a youth worker. He was planning to go to The Salvation Army training college to be an officer, to enter a lifelong ministry of helping others. I came to admire Jack's strengths and control, and I desired his love for me more than anything. Jack had swept me off my feet and that made me feel like my life was now complete.

There was a seductiveness in conceding to Jack's decisions about where we went, what we did, how we did things, and with whom. I even conceded to him the choices about the clothes I bought. Jack was making it all too easy for me not to think, under his guise or ruse of *"trust me."* I reasoned that Jack was just being helpful and caring. In giving my life and my personal power over to him, I did not know that yielding like this to him would ultimately cripple me.

2024 Spiritual Awakening:
Satan is seductive too! **He does not take our authority by force, but if we stay passive, just like Adam and Eve were in the garden of Eden, we have yielded our God-given authority to Satan. Satan then has authority over us that was never his to have!**
See Genesis 3:1-6

Now the serpent was more cunning than any beast
of the field which Yehovah GOD had made.
And he said to the woman,
"Has God indeed said,
'You shall not eat of every tree of the garden'?"
Genesis 3:1

*****

In the Gisborne summer of 1988, Jack and I married. The sunny day was beautiful, and I felt equally beautiful in the wedding gown I had made. Family and friends shared the occasion. The ceremony was full of meaning and promise. There were wedding photos on the beach and the wedding reception was in my parent's beautiful large garden.

In the first year of our married life in Christchurch, Jack was clip-boarding his way through youth ministry and I was happy at my work immersed in my nursing practice, which included health promotion and illness prevention, maternal and child health checks, wound care, diabetes care, administering immunizations, and disease management. I also syringed blocked ears and extracted perilously placed items stuck up children's noses!

As we negotiated life together, I enjoyed extending hospitality to friends and guests. I had joined Jack at The Salvation Army Corps that he and his family attended, and once again I was fully involved in Corps life. I attended the many youth events Jack was involved in or responsible for, and as Candidates for entering The Salvation Army Training College (SATC) the following year, we undertook the necessary tests and medicals and began preparations to move to Upper Hutt where the SATC was located.

As busy as we were, we took time for other outings and activities. I remember walking with Jack through Mona Vale Gardens in Christchurch. The Rhododendrons and Azaleas beautifully displaying the brilliant colors of the sunset. The dawn of my life, and the sunshine of youth had passed. I was now a young adult, a married woman, and a health professional. From dawn to sunset - little did I know what this sunset would bring. I could never have imagined what spiritual, physical and psychological battles lay ahead.

*****

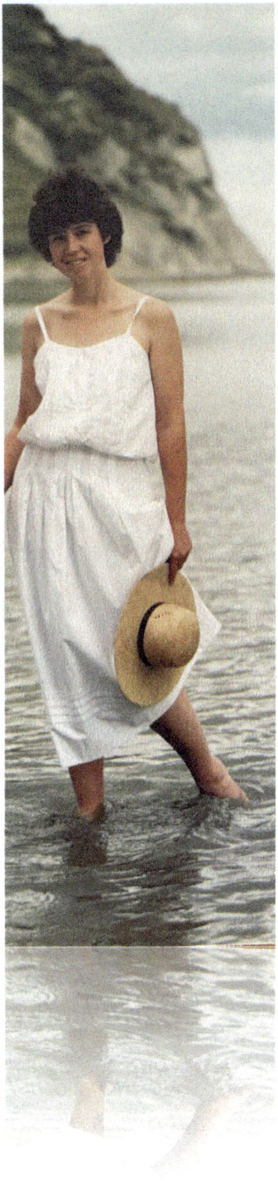

I will praise You, for ***I am fearfully and wonderfully made****;*
Marvelous are Your works,
And that my soul knows very well.
Psalm 139:14

The Sojourn

See, I have set before you today life and good, death and evil, in that I command you today to love Yehovah your God, to walk in His ways, and to keep His commandments, His statutes, and His judgments, that you may live and multiply; and Yehovah your God ***will bless you in the land which you go to possess****.*

But if your heart turns away so that you do not hear, and are drawn away, and worship other gods and serve them, I announce to you today that you shall surely perish; you shall not prolong your days in the land...
Deuteronomy 30:15-18

CHAPTER 2

Bondage In Egypt

Once he controls how she defines his abuse of her,
then he can control her actions.
And when her religious community tells her to "forgive and
keep no record of wrongs" and "as far as it is up to you,
be at peace with all men" and
"your role is to build your husband up"
... she redoubles her efforts to take responsibility
for fixing all the hurt and pain in the relationship.
As she takes this on herself, she withers
under the guilt and shame of this impossible task.
Natalie Hoffman - Is It Me?

The following year in 1989, we left Christchurch and entered The Salvation Army Training College in Upper Hutt, near Wellington, for two years of theological study and training to become officers. I believed this launch into full-time ministry together was our Heavenly Father's plan and purpose for our lives. I was twenty-five years old.

I remember that moment of trepidation, when I paused in the darkness outside the gates of The Salvation Army Training College. It had been a challenging time of preparation, and a strenuous effort to get there. I was exhausted. Our freighted belongings, which had arrived earlier that day, had been badly damaged in transit as the Pacific Freighter was battered by a fierce storm in the Cook Strait. The tail gate of the ferry had actually busted open and another truck on board had plunged into the rough seas and huge waves! Our own belongings had been flooded and almost washed into the sea as well. And so, I stood before the gates of my destiny; feeling like I too had been tossed on the raging sea. It was a sign of things to come.

For the next two years we lived on campus. There were sixteen other first year cadets and nineteen second year cadets. Our community of staff, cadets and children numbered eighty-two. The nature of life at the training college was regimented. All aspects of our lives and duties were scheduled and mandatory. Jack's coercive power and control compounded this regimentation. I continued to believe Jack was *doing good* and was *loving me*. No one had ever been so interested about me and what I did. Jack always insisted that his way of doing things was what was best for me. Although it had seemed positive in the beginning, it grew to the point of suffocating my individuality. I had given in to his control and, as a result, I was quickly losing confidence in myself. Only years later would I realize that Jack was not *doing good* and *loving me*. **His coercion and control was abuse.**

*****

As Jack's dominance grew larger, I grew smaller. I was quietly walking in his shadow, becoming a submissive reflection of what he wanted me to be. He approved my relinquishing control over my life, and it made our relationship work to his satisfaction. I still believed Jack was helping and loving me, though later I would learn that others perceived Jack's micro-management of our lives as dominating and stifling me.

From the beginning, **Jack was not recognizing me as a person but as a possession. Not as a woman to love, but a possession to be used.** And from the beginning, Jack had been mentally cataloguing me, not to love me but to manipulate and use me. This is why he was "so interested".

2024 Looking Back:
Many years later I would learn from a trauma therapist that it is not in the nature of an abuser to have an equal relationship, and that abuse is a pattern of behavior planned from the start with the intended goal to control. Abuse of any sort relies on an imbalance of power.

I realized that people who are well have independent thoughts, but right from the start of our relationship, Jack needed me to see the world exactly as he did. Jack could not tolerate me having independent thoughts. An abuser's goal is to control how you think, how you see the world, how you see everything. Because of this, I lost confidence to know that my thoughts and insights were real, true or worthwhile. What I thought to be true became untrue. What I thought to be right became wrong. Since it was Jack who was turning my thoughts upside down - I looked to Jack to validate them. From the time of meeting and dating Jack, I began to lower my boundaries and surrender my personal power to him. When Jack took my personal power, I allowed it. Submitting to my husband in this way seemed the right thing to do, yet it was to disconnect me from myself.

*****

I did well in my studies, although they were challenging. At the end of the first year, I was offered the opportunity to do post-graduate advanced theological studies. That offer was also made to Jack and two others in our cadet group. Neither Jack nor I accepted these advanced studies. I had already started to slide into anorexia. Getting to the end of the first year in college had been an endurance test and so the two-week summer holiday in December was much anticipated. It gave me the opportunity to retake some control in life, in particular, my body. With the purchase of swimming goggles and a cycling helmet I took to the water and road with discipline and determination. Physical exercise was rapidly becoming the sole part of my life that I had control over.

In January 1990, Jack and I began our second year as cadets with a three month Out-Training Appointment in Napier. This involved working one month in a social service center of The Salvation Army, and two months assisting in the local Corps. Being back in the familiar Hawkes Bay, with predictable warm sunny days and an abundance of orchard fruits, was wonderful and it soothed my soul. I enjoyed and felt comfortable in the company of those with whom we worked and socialized. The Napier Corps ministry was particularly rewarding for me.

My growing obsession for health and well-being continued within these optimal conditions. I worked hard at eating healthy and exercising. I swam almost daily, even into the colder weather, gaining energy and motivation from the power and discipline it gave me. My sense of confidence and well-being, which had been dramatically damaged, bounced back.

We returned to college in April. I was keen to get through the next eight months so as to experience a more permanent state of freedom and autonomy. This was the answer to getting my life back on track, or so I thought. What I could not face or recognize was Jack's increasing control over my life. I knew there was a problem but could not accept that allowing Jack to control my life was the cause. I had placed my security in Jack. Whenever I deferred to Jack, he took more control.

If I behaved spontaneously, such as riding my bicycle barefoot, Jack would reprimand me for being dangerously irresponsible. If I was poorly prepared for an outing I was being 'seriously careless.' Everything took on an ominous significance changing an enjoyable casual trip to the beach into a total failure of preparedness. Jack could not tolerate his own shortcomings either, but he was in control and blame or irritation was more often assigned to me. It created a deep-seated conviction in me that I was badly flawed and unable to live up to what was needed of me in our marriage.

The growing sense of being hopelessly flawed squeezed all the joy out of my life. It caused me to overreact and attempt to retake control over at least some part of my life, like eating and exercising, and led to a deep and confounding depression I could not shake. As a newlywed, I could not bring myself to see my 'loving' husband having a bearing on my increasing depression, instead, I was having continual underlying feelings of not coping because my house was not perfect. I knew that if I could work hard and make the house clean and perfect again, then I would feel more in control and be better able to handle my emotions. I realized there must be another way, but the washing, dusting, polishing, vacuuming, mopping, and wiping brought some temporary relief for me.

*****

2024 Looking Back:
Jack's need was for me to think like he did. He believed his opinions and decisions to be right, so more and more I came to believe that my opinions were wrong or unnecessary. Jack was the decision-maker because he was the one who was 'right,' and this was the reality Jack constructed.

I lost confidence in my own ability to think, choose, have an opinion and express myself. This was particularly apparent in my more unwell periods when I was in a state of free-fall. I had great difficulty discerning my needs, preferences and opinions. I certainly relied on him a great deal to speak for me, organize me, protect me from people, even choose my clothes! I believed that Jack rationalized his exerting power and control as an expression of his love for me - not as an expression of his own insecurities.

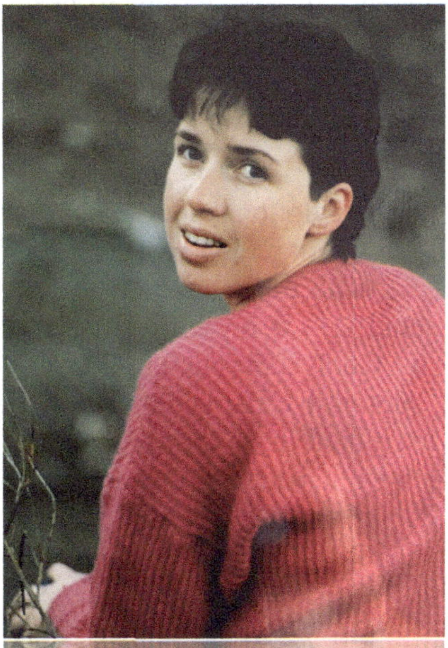

Jack's control and my acquiescing to it, was erasing my individuality and destroying my spirit. I was naive and clueless, caught up in something I could not understand, and could not recognize what it was doing to me. My parents and some Salvation Army colleagues, however, saw what I could not. It was only later, they felt free to share their observations with me.

Jack's control over my thoughts and values were perfect conditions for the sexual abuse that soon entered the marriage. I was like the frog that was put into a pot of cold water on a hot stove and the water slowly heated. The frog was unaware that she was gradually being cooked alive. And so the sexual abuse from Jack started slowly with his desire to have me wear erotic lingerie. This upset me. I protested. Wasn't sex with me good enough for Jack? Apparently, it was not. Jack was persuasive, even arguing it was needed to improve our sex life. He would lay it out upon the bed for me to wear before sex. These items were purchased by Jack. This was harmless enough I reasoned. If this was something I could do that was going to give him pleasure, then I should oblige his desire. I wanted to please him, not really daring to question his coerced desires.

Not everything that happens
in the marriage bed is sacred.
Things that are not right -
are not right in the marriage bed either!

It took me a long time to learn that sexual abuse by a husband is a form of domestic violence that can have severe physical, mental and emotional consequences for the victim. Sexual abuse in marriage violates a woman's bodily autonomy and can lead to long-lasting trauma, depression, anxiety, and post-traumatic stress disorder (PTSD). It can take many forms, including coercive sexual behavior, non-consensual (unwanted) sexual acts, sexual exploitation or objectification, unwanted intrusion of pornography or implements into sex, undesired sexual activities, and rape.

As the emotional and sexual abuse in my marriage to Jack advanced, I became more and more depressed, defeated, confused and entrapped in a state of emotionally battered submissiveness where I could not stand up for myself. There was an intense internal conflict between my Godly upbringing and the things Jack was leading me into as a "submissive wife." Something had to give in this conflict. Eventually, it erupted in anxiety, depression, anorexia and suicide attempts. The longer it went on, eventually twenty years, the more it emerged as PTSD.

*****

I obsessively embraced suggestions for a healthy and well-balanced lifestyle. Nonetheless, they sent me down a road where I overloaded myself with rules and stringent attitudes in my quest to regain control of my life. The goals I set for diet and exercise were high and ever increasing. But I was losing control over my life, and to compensate I sought ever more control over my body. I denied myself and resisted any foods that were preserved, contained fats or sugars, or seemed unnecessary. I became obsessed about checking and rechecking food to ensure I remained true to my goal of a 'pure intake.' My eating and attitudes to food soon became inflexible - refusing any food that was offered to me and often taking my own 'good' food with me when we went out.

As well as taking long walks, I swam three to four mornings a week. I was obsessed. The college day commenced at 7:30 am and so I would get up at 5:00 am to accomplish my one hundred to one hundred and fifty lengths of a local pool. The remaining mornings of the week I would cycle vigorously for at least an hour. In doing this, at first, I felt enlivened and in control of myself. Initially, praise for my discipline and resulting weight loss came readily from Jack and others. My eating and exercise became the measure of my worth. They were the only things left that I felt I could control.

2024 Looking Back:
As Jack's control was erasing my individuality and destroying my spirit, the regimentation in the Salvation Army Training College only intensified matters. I became depressed. My increasing food obsession and exercise mania were my ways of coping with this depression. The hard truth was that I now had a new Master - Satan. He had taken advantage of my weakness and loss of control by constantly feeding me lies.

As the end of training neared, and our commissioning approached, I was no longer feeling the health and fitness-thrill. My ability to cope had greatly diminished. My voice and personality, along with my desires and dreams, had shrunk smaller and smaller, practically disappearing. I lost all confidence in myself. There was a suppressed resentment that I could not admit, even to myself. I had lost eighteen kilograms (forty pounds) within the two years. I went from an ideal body weight to being skin and bones.

*****

By the time we were commissioned in January of 1991, I was living in an almost continual state of tearfulness, distress and despair - causing me to be intolerant and edgy, and feeling physically weak. I maintained my discipline, hoping against hope that I was still in control as I opposed the concerns many others expressed for my health.

A day of reckoning was bound to come and come it did. Saturday, 18 January 1991 was our commissioning day. My life with Jack was like a pressure cooker, steadily increasing in heat and pressure over the past two years until it could no longer be contained. It was about to explode and catapult me into a dark and painful journey.

**"Lieutenant Jack and Mrs Cate Campbell,
you have been appointed as
Salvation Army Corps officers to the
Dannevirke Corps."**

The edict that sounded out across the St. James theatre on the evening of our appointing - immediately put my head into a tailspin as Jack and I stood on the stage being given our appointment. How would I be able to maintain my exercise program in a place that had no year-round swimming pool? My mind searched frantically to work it out. Perhaps I could travel to the swimming pools at Palmerston North? Maybe I could get an Exercycle? I was desperate. What should have evoked in me the joy and expectation of embarking on our calling into ministry was drowned in panic.

Jack and I made our final departure from The Salvation Army Officer Training College on a very hot mid-January day in 1991 to take up our first appointment as Corps officers in the small town of Dannevirke. Our small Ford Lazer car was once again being used more like a truck than a car. We had used every available nook and cranny to take the smaller and more delicate items we had not packed onto the removal truck.

My precious African violet plants I could not have on my lap or at my feet had been carefully placed on the parcel tray at the back of the car. The journey from Upper Hutt to Dannevirke took only three hours, but with the temperature over 30°C (86°F), it seemed longer. Arriving at our Dannevirke quarters, I was mortified to find the beautifully flowering African violet plants on the car's parcel tray, the ones I had propagated from leaves, were severely suffering from heat exhaustion and burns. As we travelled, they had not only been exposed to the direct sun, but the hatch window had intensified the heat. I feared these plants were beyond reviving. I had no choice but to put a few of these African violet plants 'to rest.' I felt as wilted as the violets.

Certain conditions were needed for these plants to do well— light and porous soil, an even, warm and dry temperature, minimal watering, good light, but not direct sunshine. In the following months of summer and autumn, the condition of some of the remaining African violet plants improved and became stable, but the recovery I had hoped for did not come, despite my best efforts to nurture them back to health and vitality. Then came a cold winter, living in a cold house. So even if these African violet plants were kept warm during the day when the room was heated, they had to survive the chilling night temperatures. Consequently, some of my plants struggled to live. Just like the African violets - people need the right conditions to thrive.

The discovery of two trees in our back yard laden with apples and nectarines somewhat soothed my distress. In fact, the fruit trees, and the grape hyacinths and freesias that surprisingly emerged in spring, turned out to be the only pleasurable memories I have of Dannevirke.

As a newly commissioned Lieutenant, I had endeavored to fulfill my role as a Salvation Army Corps officer— visiting Corps congregants, leading children's Sunday school, playing the piano (very badly) for Sunday services, and sharing the preaching ministry with Jack, but I was becoming more and more fragile in body and mind.

'Burn-out' is not an unusual happening for persons in 'people' orientated professions, but it doesn't happen just weeks out of the gate! Why was I falling apart and unable to cope with the simplest of responsibilities? To face people was a hard enough task, let alone lead a women's or children's group. I was losing my grip.

I saw an incredible likeness between my African violet plants that were struggling for life and my struggle for life. I wrote in my journal of feeling like one particular African violet plant of mine, which had become unsightly and an embarrassment because of its depleted form. Even in the most suitable environment our house could offer, its growth was stunted, the leaves were in bad condition, the soil was sodden and heavy, and there was certainly no likelihood of bloom. I referred to this plant by my own name. It was not suitable to be displayed in the living room, kitchen or even the main bedroom. Should it be banished to the spare bedroom with the door shut where no one would see it? Put outside? Why not just throw it out? I decided to keep this 'Cate' plant in the spare room that was continually cold and damp until I could make a more definite decision about its destiny.

I felt a certain abandonment. It was as if, like my ‘Cate’ plant, I had been shoved out on the back step, exposed to all the intensity of the elements - sun, wind, heat, cold and frost. All security and protection gone. Each day I was made aware of yet another thing that I was unable to cope with. With each realization, a brown wizened leaf dropped. Very few leaves were now left.

Due to my dramatic weight loss, Jack took me to a doctor, at his mother’s urging. The doctor told me that I did not have a problem. It was pleasing for me to hear I had no problem, and that all I needed to do was to eat as much of anything that I liked! This seemed to satisfy Jack, and was a useful opinion to pacify concerned friends and family - my critics - for a time. In truth, I was continually stressed out about my weight. My unexpressed intention was to keep reducing my food intake, which I did. And so it was, that in our first year of being Salvation Army officers I was put on sick leave.

Being in Dannevirke for such a short time had not given me the opportunity to establish friendships or develop a support system and so our call for help went out to a couple in Palmerston North whom we knew a little, and were also Salvation Army Officers. Ed had recently come through a burn-out experience, and Patricia seemed like an understanding sort of person. I remember telling her one evening that my difficulties *"seem so simple but feel so complicated."* The road between Dannevirke and Palmerston North became very familiar to us over that year. We made frequent visits to Ed and Patricia's home. They were my lifeline.

More importantly, I also began to see a counselor (who was also a medical doctor) in Palmerston North, who diagnosed me as having Anorexia Nervosa. Coming to terms with the diagnosis of anorexia from Dr. Andy Stone did not happen easily or immediately for me. I would not allow Jack to use the word in my presence and certainly made it hard for him to be honest with others who were concerned. Eventually however, I got past the denial.

*****

2024 Looking Back:
According to the Emily Project, eating disorders impact about 30 million people in the United States. These disorders include Anorexia Nervosa, Bulimia Nervosa, and Binge-Eating Disorder.

Eating disorders are serious conditions related to persistent eating behaviors that negatively impact an individual's health, emotions, and ability to function in important areas of life. Most eating disorders involve focusing too much on weight, body shape and food, leading to dangerous eating behaviors.

A study from JAMA Psychiatry on suicide and eating disorders found that the risk for a suicide attempt is markedly higher among individuals with an eating disorder. These individuals often experience intense suffering, feeling like their pain, hopelessness, depression or self-hated will never end and so seek a way to escape overwhelming emotions. Their need for help should be taken seriously.

Anorexia Nervosa is characterized by weight loss, intense fear of gaining weight, and a distorted perception of weight and shape. Individuals with anorexia will excessively limit calories or use other methods to lose weight, such as excessive exercise, using laxatives or diet aids, or vomiting after eating.

Anorexia Nervosa has the highest mortality rate of any psychological disorder!

This is due to the numerous medical complications that accompany it, and the very real danger of suicide. Up to 20% of those with anorexia attempt suicide, and as many as 43% report suicidal ideation. Individuals with anorexia are nine times more likely than non-anorexic peers to attempt suicide.

Studies cited by the American Association of Suicidology (*Holm-Denoma et al, 2008; Kaye, 2008; Keel et al., 2003*) indicate that the suicide mortality rate of people with anorexia is one of the highest of all psychiatric illnesses.

Even more disturbing is the intensity of anorexia sufferers' suicide attempts. *Holm-Denoma et al.* found that when individuals with anorexia decide to end their life, they typically use highly lethal methods, indicating they truly wish to kill themselves and aren't just sending out a cry for help.

Research has shown those with eating disorders often present with a second disorder such as substance abuse, anxiety, trauma, or depression. That is why it is so important that every disorder a person is experiencing is treated during eating disorder treatment.

Without treatment, up to 20 percent of sufferers with a serious eating disorder will die!

2024 Spiritual Awakening:

And the sons of Israel went to buy grain
among those who journeyed,
for famine was in the land of Canaan.
Genesis 42:5

Although Judah and his household were living in Canaan, the land promised to the Israelites, it was not yet theirs. They were sojourners in the land under the authority of Canaanite kings. Even then, Yehovah had foreseen the need of His people. Even before the famine, Yehovah sent Joseph ahead, through trial and tribulation, to be the answer to their needs.

When a disease that kills 20% of its sufferers is upon us, Yehovah will provide answers. Yehovah has allowed trials and tribulations in my life to equip me to bring help to others.

The secondary and pre-existing disorder I had with anorexia was depression which related to my marriage with Jack. Another secondary disorder of anxiety was later to emerge.

Dr. Lerner, clinical psychologist, says it's important to pay attention to whether an individual has a condition that predates the eating disorder, such as depression, as eating disorders have a high occurrence of co-morbidities. In these cases, the issues regarding the eating disorder may be resolved, but the preexisting condition will continue or possibly worsen, particularly if the eating disorder helped a patient cope with the original condition.

*****

During that endless year in Dannevirke I became quite expert at playing 'hide and seek'. Unlike the child who plays 'hide and seek' to have fun, I played it in all seriousness. For me, the game was motivated by fear and shame. I would hide from people known and unknown if I suspected the threat of examining eyes or a conversation. It seemed to me that I was less than whole by nature and by appearance, and that this was plainly obvious to anyone. As much as I hated the aloneness of living in a place that was unfamiliar and without support, it seemed to be the place I deserved.

Dannevirke was a small town, and like most small towns, most people know most things about most everyone. I therefore strategically timed my walks for when the main populace had not yet woken, or in the dark of night. When I had to get in the car Jack would signal an 'all-clear' so as to avoid our curious neighbors who were frequently hanging over the fence. I would avoid answering the telephone and door at all costs. Not that the telephone was too much of a problem as Jack was quick to purchase an answer-phone. This meant I could screen telephone calls, only answering Jack or Patricia. Patricia rang me most days.

Ignoring and avoiding house-callers however, was not always so easily managed and I would freeze in fear when someone knocked on the door. It was bad enough having to conceal myself from the front door-knockers, but I dreaded those back door-knockers the most - as the dining room windows provided little obscurity and the kitchen windows gave absolutely none! It also seemed to me, in my paranoid imagination, that a few regular callers made it their business to know what was going on at the Salvation Army house.

One morning soon after Jack had gone out for a short time, a tradesman came to the door. He was a back-door-knocker, but fortunately (or so I thought) I was in the bedroom when he declared his presence. Much to my relief he left, having knocked several times with no response. Just moments later though, a blue and white car came roaring up to the house. A policeman then identified himself as he entered our house through the unlocked door.

Well I knew I had not committed any crimes that the police would be concerned with! So instead of being busted in my own house, I decided to reveal myself. The cop was confused when I told him there was no problem, that I lived there, and I had not left the house all morning. He had received a report that someone was present in the house, seen beside an open window in one of the bedrooms. The informant had assumed that this person should not have been there as they would not answer the door.

Then there was the time when a vagrant visited our house. Our house was identified as belonging to The Salvation Army, so this was where people might come for help. Again, Jack was out, but on this occasion he was away for a few hours. First of all, this destitute looking character knocked on the front door. I did my usual freeze, fully expecting that he would soon take his leave when he realized the house was unoccupied. But he did not. Instead, he tried the back door, then the front door again, then the back door again, and the front door again until he was duly assured that no one in The Salvation Army house was there to assist him.

Then, to my unexpected horror, he set up camp on our front doorstep, just a meter away from where I stood. Until then I had dared not move a muscle due to our badly squeaky floors which would have given me away for sure. Now I *definitely* could not attempt my usual crawling to safety under the window height as I was standing on a particularly squeaky section.

I do not think my terrorized facial expression changed a millimeter throughout the ordeal, but I suppose things did get better. After the immediate terror and panic of my dilemma, my stressed limbs relaxed, (about half an hour later) and I assumed an easier squatting pose. There I continued to wait in anguish for ten centuries until Jack rescued me. Time passed slowly. I was a shattered bundle of nerves by the time Jack finally arrived home - much later than expected - and took care of helping the man in need!

In retrospect, I think my Dannevirke year can claim credit for heightening those senses that served to protect me from real and perceived threats. My ears became vigilantly attuned to hearing footsteps and voices. I developed radar eyes that could spy a familiar person across a crowded shop or 50 meters down the road and so change track to avoid contact. I was able to sniff out foods and know how to avoid eye contact with them. As for my sense of touch, well I generally hated that. I was resistant to having others touch me as it was like having my 'fat' button pressed. At the time I thought people did this to upset me.

'Taste' was the only sense that must have deteriorated. In that year I made an extreme transition from consuming only the purest food forms to episodes of bingeing on foods that were on my 'bad' list. Not only this, but often what I ate would not have been at all palatable to most people in its raw or frozen state. It was as if I had to eat it in a degraded state to ease my shame.

I did not cope well with loud noise and lots of people, and so avoided such scenes. Living continually on edge made me very jumpy. I was a frustrating back-seat driver to Jack. I certainly did not attempt to drive the car myself for quite some time. I was even too nervous to cross a street or board an escalator without clutching Jack. My appreciation of beauty and beautiful things was greatly diminished, as to see and experience such things was to have my 'ugly,' 'worthless,' and 'shameful' buttons pressed all at once. I also became increasingly unable to cope with simple domestic tasks which I had always enjoyed and done well.

Once a week I would go to see Dr. Andy. At the time it was difficult to identify the cause of the anorexia. I had not suffered with anorexia or any other mental illness in my life prior to marriage, and I insisted Jack was a 'devoted' husband.

Therefore, the focus gravitated to my childhood, assuming the causative issues lay there. The problem with this therapy perspective, was that my parents were not the problem. They never had been the problem! They were good parents - and my childhood and teenage years were good and sound. Although I had a quiet personality, I grew up to be confident, enterprising and independent. Nonetheless, the 'parental problem' remained the focus of my therapy over nearly twenty years.

2024 Looking Back:
There was never any earnest attempt by mental health professionals to look at Jack's power and control in the marriage. I am amazed that experienced mental health professionals throughout my many years of psychiatric care were not better detectives. If I had been murdered, my husband would have been the prime suspect, regardless of how he and others professed his innocence. Yet there seemed to be no

suspicion or awareness that Anorexia Nervosa could have developed because of emotional or sexual abuse in a marriage. The parents were the traditional culprits.

The year in Dannevirke was a period of identity crisis that struck me suddenly and severely. My 'disguise' was ripped off, leaving me naked, degraded, shamed, worthless, and confused.

There were a number of noticeable changes recognized by others. One was the clothes I chose to wear. For most of my life I had worn dresses and skirts in preference to trousers. Dresses were conservative and 'nice,' as were the rest of my clothes. This changed dramatically when in January 1991, I began to think of myself as too fat to wear dresses - they were too prissy and ‘nice' anyway. They were the 'old Cate' who sat nicely, tidily and compliantly. The 'old Cate' I did not want to be anymore!

My black pants, big baggy black jersey and boots were pretty much all I wore. I went into hiding. I was not a nice person, and I did not want to look nice. I dressed like this because it was extreme and painted me black to others who often were unsure of me and distanced themselves. Black was the way I felt about myself ,so it was appropriate.

I rejected not only my familiar soft pastel colors that were safe, conservative, and pretty - but all colors - other than black that is. Not only the colors of clothes, but I also rejected the colors of decor, art, and food. At best I would tolerate their presence. Maybe this was why I was so often reduced to tears in my 'black' times when I was over-awed by a concentrated abundance of color. What I finally came to appreciate were bold, strong, and distinct colors, textures and lines.

Being the 'good' Christian that I was, meant that my speech had always been pure. I had accepted that others could swear, and speak crudely and discourteously, but not me. My language suddenly became not so 'virginal.' As well as the frustration and despair I was experiencing, there was also the new emotion of anger to cope with. My 'nice' words were not adequate or suitable as I attempted to express my innermost anguish.

My attitude and response to music was another thing that changed. Contemporary Christian music and brass band music had been a big part of my life. For almost the whole year I was in Dannevirke, I could not bear to listen to music of any kind - especially Christian music!

I declared my 'change' further when I had my hair shaved off. This evidenced my desperation and wish to be rejected. I was never sure if I really liked it that way, as much as I tried to convince myself and others. However I was sure that I did not want to look like I once had.

Starving myself and exercising excessively had resulted in me not having a regular monthly cycle for two years. I had a *love~hate* relationship with food. I was always thinking about it. How to assess, avoid, restrict, hide, deny, view, smell, touch, steal, binge and 'reverse.' I dreamed about food and cooking, even how to feed others. I obsessively collected and hoarded recipes, without ever using them. These thoughts were rarely peaceful or pleasant. Much anguish and mental torment was often observable to those in my company. These thoughts translated themselves into behaviors that were frequently shameful and punishing.

My body weight was an unceasing concern for me. To my way of thinking, eating food meant an instant and visible deposit of fat on my body. The mirrors in our house mocked and tormented me about my fat and failure, yet I relied on them to judge and berate my body. Shop windows and mirrors did little to bring pleasure or harmony to any excursion I made!

The bathroom scale and I privately met ritualistically every morning. I was not always courteous to it and often held it in contempt when it didn't show me an acceptable number. Other times it was a rewarding ally. The scale was well travelled because where I went, it went! When I look at my bathroom scale today, I remember the times it was kicked, sworn at, and hidden from me.

The type of clothes I wore not only reflected my depressed mood, but also reflected my distorted body-image. This was more of an issue to others than myself. To me, my weight was too excessive to wear skirts or dresses even if I had wanted to. My one pair of trousers and a big baggy jersey were monotonous but a camouflaging comfort. There did come a time though when I began to be more daring. This started one day when I purchased two more pairs of trousers and another jersey. I would engage in lengthy and tiring internal debate as I dressed before a mirror - often changing numerous times before feeling assured that I was sufficiently hidden.

My mind was acutely attuned to messages that I perceived as being a judgement on my weight. I would resist buying a bottle of shampoo from a supermarket shelf if it had 'extra body' on the label. To see an excessively overweight person eating a cream bun or pie was like seeing a mirror image of myself. In panic, I would adhere even more rigorously to my food limits and restrictions. If someone told me I was 'looking better,' I translated this to mean that they thought I was fatter than when they last saw me.

The other obsessive-compulsive tactics that I used to reduce weight seemed to have no real effect. Perhaps they were only guilt-relievers for the sin of eating. At the time I was convinced that they were necessary and effective. Such things as drinking vinegar in the hope that it would break-down my body fat, or allowing myself to be cold so that my fat would be punished and shivered away. It was not only in the bingeing phases that excessive laxative use and throwing up kept my stomach feeling acceptably empty. At one stage I was 'reversing' four or five times a day after eating the most insignificant amounts. To get even close to feeling full was frightening and guilt-inducing.

I was experiencing the pendulum swing between starving and bingeing. The pendulum was in a continual state of motion between the extremes that were overpowering and demoralizing. I did not understand what was causing me to lose myself and bring about this demise of my mental health.

I ended up paying dearly for losing myself in this illness, causing grave physical, mental, emotional and spiritual devastation. I reasoned that discovering the truth about myself, God and my relationships with others, was all-important to me. Everything in my life was being scrutinized to see if I wanted to keep it, toss it, or change it.

At the beginning of our two years in The Salvation Army Training College I weighed 70 kilograms (154 pounds). This was within the ideal weight range for my build and height of 1.79 meters (5 foot 10 inches). By the time we graduated my weight had dropped to 54 kilograms (119 pounds). Six months later I was 46 kilograms (101 pounds). I had lost 53 lbs, one third of my body weight! Even at this weight I was convinced of my obesity. In fact, the lower my weight became, the more obese I believed myself to be. The disease was a demon that drove me ever harder. I was at war with myself!

Thursday 28 March 1991

I saw Dr. Andy yesterday. He tells me that God wants the African violet plant dead. He states that God is neither embarrassed with, disappointed with, or indifferent to the plant. Dr. Andy suggests that God is taking extra special care of this plant in His special plant nursery. He is speaking to me as a child. Death comes before rebirth. I already feel dead.

Friday 29 March 1991

I do not care how much weight I lose, but always in the back of my mind is the question, 'will this stop me from becoming pregnant?' Still, if I cannot become pregnant, and it certainly seems that way, why not take up the challenge and see how thin I can get. What does it matter anyway!

Monday 1 April 1991

Today is the first time I can’t trust myself. I feel like I could do harm to myself. These thoughts are overpowering me.

Thursday 4 April 1991

Jack asks me if I really want to change. I don’t know how and the effort is too much. It’s easier to keep stumbling down to a final end. To give up.

Tuesday 9 April 1991

Jack's questions are too big and vague which makes them difficult to answer. He also responds to my answers in a threatening and corrective way. Despite Jack's efforts, I feel more alone at home because he can’t reach me or identify with me. I don’t think I trust him anymore. Do I still even love him?

2024 Looking Back:
I believe that at this point Jack felt he was in over his head with me. He had created a monster he could not contain.

Wednesday 17 April 1991
The past few days have been desperate - sinking lower and lower. I cannot believe that people can love or care for me. I want to die. I am not worth their time or concern. I hate going to bed at night. Too many hours of darkness, aloneness, quietness and sleeplessness that pass so slowly. Too much time to think of suicide. It's scary. I am scared!

Tuesday 23 April 1991
I am waking most mornings with a headache. Is it from not sleeping or from not eating? Both, no doubt.

Wednesday 1 May 1991
Where has all this anger within me come from? I don't know how to handle it. Yesterday Jack and I bought a duvet, but when we got home I didn't like it. My anger erupted. I was angry with the duvet and with our house that needs countless improvements. I was angry with our situation. I was angry with me. I was angry at Jack! Throwing my shoes at him and hitting the wall brought no measure of relief to the all-consuming anger trapped inside me.

Sunday 5 May 1991
Jack has bought me a doughnut ring cushion as my emaciated tail bone is extremely sore when sitting, especially traveling in the car.

Tuesday 21 May 1991
I was really angry last night because Jack went out and was away a lot longer than expected. In response, I took to the Exercycle and fiercely cycled another 25 kilometers (15.5 miles). My body felt close to death.

Saturday 1 June 1991
I will admit to no one that my hands and feet are numb, my heart is frequently palpitating and my mouth is ulcerated. I am spending lots of time in bed, especially in the evenings, as it is a place without

expectations, and it is away from food. It is also a place of comfort and warmth for me.

Eating disorder recovery can be difficult when it
takes place outside an eating disorder treatment center.
It requires multidisciplinary treatment due to medical complications,
dietary needs, and psychological needs.
Michael Rollin, MD, Psychiatrist
Eating Disorder Center of Denver

Sunday 23 June 1991
A letter from Jack to my parents, telling them to stay away:

13 June 1991

Dear Mum and Dad,

I am sure that in time, you and other family members will be included in Cate's world, but at the moment it is too much for her. You would not think she was performing, but then nobody has before.

So I suppose the thing we have to ask is, can you put aside the frustration and hurt, and try to understand what I have written (or at least accept it) for the benefit of Cate? It really is the only way she will, and is getting better. There is no element of wanting to hurt anyone!

Please continue to ring, write and pray. We do want to keep contact, but just not physically at the moment. Of course there will be some things that are very personal to Cate, which I will not be able to talk about with you. I really do hope this letter is of help.

Jack

Saturday 29 June 1991
I took another thirty laxatives, having already had my usual twenty this morning. I felt like I was going to die. Of course I couldn't tell Jack what I'd done.

Mirror, mirror on the wall

Sunday 30 June 1991
Sometimes for a split second I feel thin. Then I look in a mirror or touch myself, and the distressing realization comes again that I am disgustingly fat. People are talking nonsense when they say I am underweight. I can only image that their words are intended to make me feel better. Well they don't!

Tuesday 2 July 1991
I tried on a pair of jeans in Palmerston North yesterday. My immediate response was that they were great, especially at just $39.00. Jack came into the fitting room and said he thought they looked good on me too. Then the mirror suddenly changed, showing me as fat and ugly! In an instant I was overwhelmed by self-hatred. This was obvious to Jack. I was then hostile and angry, making it difficult for Jack to reason with me.

Is what I saw first the deception, and what I saw second the truth? Or was it the other way around, as Jack tried to have me believe? He persuaded me to go with my first response, that the jeans looked good on me. We bought the jeans. I won't wear them with anything but my big black jersey.

Both female and male anatomy are disturbing to me. I hate my own with its lumps and bumps, and the male form - which Jack merely represents - is increasingly troubling to me.

2024 Looking Back:
It is easy now to see that my distorted body image, was the work of Satan, the enemy of our souls.

The thief, Satan, comes to steal and kill and destroy; I, Yeshua, have come that they may have life *and have it to the full.*
John 10:10

The untrue and perverted perception of myself that Satan caused me to see, was a massive deception that I fell for. When suffering with anorexia, Satan attempted to destroy the truth of who I was, what I looked like, and my very life! He did not want me to see myself the way my loving Abba-Yehovah created me and saw me, or for me to fulfill my God-given destiny. This was not to be the only trick Satan would pull on me in the years to come, creating a perverted perception of myself.

First and foremost, [anorexia] is a severe mental illness that takes over peoples' lives. It not only takes over their behavior but their physical health and the content of their minds. One of the biggest frustrations of people with eating disorders is that it's what they spend their day thinking about, planning around, and essentially doing all day long. It hijacks their lives and in that way, they often feel like they have no respite.

Michael Rollin, MD, Psychiatrist
Eating Disorder Center of Denver

*****

Thursday 4 July 1991
Yesterday Jack discovered there was less money in my purse than there should have been. I am sure he suspected, and quite rightly so, that I had purchased more laxatives. This led to a big argument about honesty and truthfulness.

Friday 12 July 1991
I have no desire for sex. I have no interest in it and am obviously distressed when Jack wants it. Jack says he feels like he is raping me

each time we have sex. Sex is infrequent and Jack complains that we will soon be sleeping in separate beds. He is not happy. Neither am I.

I wear clothes to bed as I feel less exposed and threatened. It's bad enough *feeling* my fat body without *seeing* it and having it *seen*.

Monday 22 July 1991

Jack's frustration and anger is often vented at me in his 'let me talk some sense into you sessions.' I then feel like I have been screwed into the ground. He talks so much, so fast, and so long, that when he asks me to respond - I can't! There's no way I can assimilate everything. Today in one of these 'sessions' he said that if things do not show significant improvement, there is no way he could accept any future appointment. That we would be forced to resign.

2024 Looking Back:

I came to think of these times as 'brow beating sessions.' I hated these regular sessions when Jack would critique me or beat out an issue. Once we had children, Jack would have these brow beating sessions with me in our bedroom. He would close the door, sometimes blocking it so the children could not enter or interrupt. When Jack was full on with me, I'd feel like I had to batten down the hatches to protect myself. The experience of being regularly brow beaten is deeply engraved upon my memory.

These intense conversations with Jack wearied me to the depths of my soul. Jack would grow increasingly frustrated or angry at not getting the responses from me that he wanted. I felt battered, confused and depressed, often to the point of paralysis. It was a trauma to my spirit. I almost always needed to sleep after these sessions. And I did. Shutting down under the covers was a safe place to withdraw. At this point the children would be told, *"Mum is sleeping now."* These sessions happened multiple times every week.

Tuesday 23 July 1991

I am scared to get better. I cannot believe that the resulting change would be lasting, authentic and radical enough. Maybe I am being stubborn, but not to the degree, or for the reasons that Jack thinks. I need to prove to Jack that things are getting better. But how?? If I knew, wouldn't I be doing it?

I frequently hear him say on the telephone to others that encouraging things are happening, but all he seems to tell me is that they are not! Is he telling them what they want to hear? What does he believe? I know it is hard for him and unfair that he should bear so much strain. He says he would never leave me. That if we split-up it would be because I left him. Yet I look at Jack and hear the emotions now frequently being expressed, and think he is very close to leaving me to sort out my own mess.

I feel like everyone significant in our lives is against me. That they are all on Jack's side. I feel so desperately alone in my world. Even God is unable or unwilling to penetrate the bubble I pathetically exist in. I see myself separated from society. Living in my own world. It is a predicament I can not change.

Wednesday 24 July 1991
Food - does not really matter to me how it tastes. I do not feel deserving of nice things anyway. The inevitable conclusion of this activity leaves my insides strained and pained. This is no 'tunnel' experience as some suggest to me. It is a big black lonely pit without means of escape.

Tuesday 30 July 1991
I was a cocktail mix of nervousness, fear, distress, aggression and pain, as I boarded the Christchurch-bound flight yesterday. I am staying a couple of weeks with Barry and Patricia - college friends, for support and a change of scenery.

I've decided I will find a hairdresser and have them shave my hair off. Maybe I should have gone to the *'Curl Up & Dye'* hair salon in Palmerston North!

Thursday 1 August 1991
The hairdresser seemed quite surprised and was very unsure when I asked her to shave my hair off to a 'number one' - to leave me with just a couple of millimeters. It seemed to take forever before she stopped asking questions like: *"You're really sure you want this?" "Why?" "Does anyone know?"* - What business was it of hers? Finally, she got on with the job. Part way through, in an attempt to

make me, or her, feel better, she said, *"you can do a lot of things with a 'number-one'."* That was weird.

Saturday 3 August 1991

The *we love you and care about you* messages are empty words to me. Today Jack's mother was highly emotional about me not believing that she loved me. "Even if you had ten heads and orange hair," she said, "we would still love you." I guess this also meant no hair! She seemed more distressed than I am. If that's even possible.

2024 Looking Back:

I had a great many letters, cards and flowers sent to me during this time. I was very disbelieving of their kind and caring words, particularly the *"we love you"* words. It was impossible for me to comprehend that in my pathetic state of being, I could be loved.

I frequently reflected back on our commissioning weekend when Jack and I became Salvation Army officers. It was a big occasion that was shared by family and friends. My dominant memories of that intense weekend were the desperate feelings I had of trying to keep myself together, and the continual comments made to me, and about me, of my appearance. At the time, I interpreted people's concern about my under-weight body as criticisms.

Monday 5 August 1991

I have two voices in my head. One voice is the 'denying' Cate who is strong-willed and disciplined. The other voice is the 'over-indulging' Cate who looks at every bit of food in sight and covets it. These conflicting voices give me no peace in my lonely world.

Thursday 10 October 1991

I feel so tired of trying. The struggle is so constant. How long will the grace of God extend to me? Will Jack's patience run out? Jack has said that it could destroy our marriage.

Saturday 12 October 1991

Patricia asked me some time ago why I seem so attracted to dominant personality types. Am I? I don't know. I went for a walk with Jack last night. He was down and disgruntled. He does not know where we are headed. I feel panic inside. I am messing up his life as well as my own. I should just "snap out of it," "buck myself up." If only I could go to bed and never again wake up. My problems would end, and Jack could start over.

Wednesday 16 October 1991
I have become obsessed with jigsaw puzzles. I do them every day. My life seems like a giant jigsaw puzzle with pieces missing that I can't ever find.

The intense anger I experienced a few months ago is back. I feel angry at Jack, food and things. I feel angry at me. Sunday afternoon was a bad time. In an attempt to relieve this all-consuming emotion, I deliberately wrecked the jigsaw I had been working on for the past two weeks. Of the 1000 pieces, there had only been a dozen left to place.

If I thought this destructive act disturbed Jack, he was even more disturbed after I punched him! I then lay on the bedroom floor sobbing uncontrollably. Jack had no idea what to do to calm or comfort me, and he sat with an expression of utter helplessness and despondency on his face.

Jack salvaged the messed-up jigsaw pieces as best he could. I just wanted it out of my sight and to try and forget about it. Jack was more lucid and settled by this stage and suggested that I decide later. I got up early this morning to re-form and finish the jigsaw. The last few days I have gone back to bed in the afternoon in utter despair and disgust with myself.

I told Dr. Andy how Jack was not being, or was not able to be, the friend I needed. That he was a lecturer, rebuker and drill sergeant - but not a friend.

Friday 18 October 1991
Things went downhill yesterday afternoon again when Jack was out. I made an attack on cereal and banana, sausages, biscuits and finished it

off with Jack's ice-cream. The inevitable feelings followed the inevitable 'reversal.'

Jack encouraged me to go out for a walk which was long and silent. We ended up sitting in the grandstand at the sports ground and we began to talk. I told him that I knew no reason to get better other than that I should for him and The Salvation Army. Jack agreed that these reasons alone are not enough - that I had to want to get better for myself.

Monday 4 November 1991

Jack drove me down to Upper Hutt yesterday afternoon. I am staying a few days with Rebekah and Richard as a result of the desperateness of Saturday. My eating had been totally out of control while Jack spent the day clearing out the garage. After two major bingeing and reversing episodes, I was worn out in every sense of the word. In a traumatized state I got myself into the shower to make some attempt at purifying myself. Here I screamed and sobbed. I had lost my sanity.

Jack had come in at this stage and helped me out of the shower. He didn't know what to do. He ended up taking a car-load of rubbish to the dump. On his return, he found me just as had left me, standing undried and clenching a towel in my hand. I was in a catatonic state and so could not talk or move. I had had enough. It was a turning point of sorts.

Saturday 9 November 1991

I've come to Auckland to have a respite with my friends, Frank and Milly. I came up with Patricia who is staying with her grandmother.

I hate this world! It is so busy - too busy to care. Everyone around me, everyone who could possibly be of any help is too busy. This world is so complicated. The more I think, the more I hurt and realize the pointlessness of life. Why live for the sake of busyness? There are so many conflicts within me: eat or not eat, truth or deception, honesty or lies, hope or hopelessness. But my greatest conflict is between LIFE and DEATH.

Eating disorders have one of the highest mortality rates in comparison to other psychiatric illnesses, and 1 in 5 individuals with anorexia nervosa who die, do so due to suicide. Furthermore, people with an eating disorder are more likely to engage in self-harm and experience suicidal ideation.
mqmentalhealth.org

I do not want to live, but I am not sure if I want to kill myself. I had hoped that Patricia would run the car off the road yesterday as we drove to Auckland. That way I would not be responsible for ending my life. I feel so desperately unhappy. It is an unhappiness no one can reach. I feel pain, but only for friends and family if I die. Otherwise, I am trapped in a numbed silent state of depression.

Today I found a load of painkillers in Frank and Milly's kitchen cupboard.

The world I had created for myself was not only isolated and black but silent!

*****

Soon after arriving at Frank and Milly's home, I had got up at 6:00 am and walked to the Henderson pools in the rain. I swam badly for an hour. This was my first swim since March, and I felt like a novice. I stayed in my bedroom all afternoon while Frank and Milly's daughter Stacey had her 9th birthday party. Suicidal thoughts had overtaken my mind. I wanted only to die.

Late afternoon Frank and Milly summoned me to the lounge to do some serious talking. Well, it was really to give me an ear bashing as they spoke harshly about having to 'buck myself up,' 'start wanting to get well,' 'stop having people on.' Frank continued by saying *"I will pray in every way for your wellness, but I will not lose any sleep over you. I will sleep soundly tonight because I am certain that your suicide thoughts amount to nothing."*

It was at this point I said to Frank, *"I want to say that I hate you. Not because I do hate you, but because hate is the strongest word I know. If I could find an equally strong word that expressed the anger and annoyance I feel about your ignorant and 'all-knowing' manner, I would use it!"* I returned to my bedroom where both Frank and Milly came in separately and expressed to me their love and concern in a much gentler and kinder manner.

The self-loathing associated with anorexia is so punishing that extreme measures might be taken to end that suffering.
Connie Quinn, DSW, LCSW-R,
Director: The Renfrew Center of New York

I had previously planned to overdose the next morning while the family was at church, but as the two children had gone to spend the night with grandparents and Frank and Milly were attending a 21st birthday party, that night seemed more opportune. Why exist through more hours of misery than I had to? Frank and Milly's answer to my problem might have worked if I was anyone else. I felt worthless. I would have gotten myself together by now if I could have! And so for them to call 'chin up' to me from the safety of the shore as I was drowning was a heartless insult.

I deserve to die!

Patricia had told me earlier in the day that she would ring me during the evening to check if I was okay. This was a threat to my plan. So once Frank and Milly had left, I was about to enact my plan when Patricia rang via a pre-arranged code. I was both angry and panicked by this interruption. I knew I had to answer her call, because she would come over straight away if I did not.

I had tried to make it sound to Patricia like I was okay, and that I was doing better than when she had seen me that morning. She was quite unconvinced. Patricia told me that our mutual friend, Beth, was also planning to ring me that evening. I asked Patricia if she would get Beth to ring me tomorrow as I was having an early night and did not feel like talking. Patricia simply said that Beth's decision to ring or not ring was hers. I guess Patricia wanted Beth to ring me. And she did!

The fifteen-minute conversation with Beth seemed like fifty. Patricia rang a second time and asked me what I was doing. She did not seem to believe me when I told her I was off to bed. Apparently, Patricia had rung Ed and Jack a couple of times that day expressing her concern for me. Being reasonably sure that Patricia's interrogation calls had ended, I took the hundred painkiller tablets I had stashed. I knew this was an ample number to finish me. It was a cold night, and so I wrapped myself in a blanket.

Anorexia Nervosa & Suicide

Suicide attempts in patients with anorexia nervosa are somewhat common. Attempts are typically serious and with an intention to die. Of those with anorexia nervosa who attempted suicide, 78% wanted to die during their attempt and 56% thought they would die. Those with anorexia nervosa binging and purging subtype (AN-BP) are at an increased risk of suicide compared to those with the restricting subtype (AN-R).
World Health Organization 2020
World report on violence and health

*****

Frank and Milly later found me in a semi-conscious state. I remember being pounded on the chest incessantly by the ambulance attendants, and then at the hospital I had some awareness of having my clothes ripped off. I had my stomach pumped and a carbonized antidote was administered to further rid my body of the medication. I was brought to consciousness as I spewed my way through the early morning hours. This was the most unloved, unlovable, and lonely that I had ever felt!

Each time I violently heaved up the black revolting stuff I was incontinent, yet I was too ill and doped up to gain control over the situation. How degraded, disgusted and wrecked I felt. I was, and remained, angry with myself for making my pain worse. I had not thought it was possible to be in worse pain!

Patricia had arrived at the hospital early Sunday morning and spent the whole day with me. Jack arrived mid-morning. The medical ward was distressing for me, however I did appreciate the many undeserved expressions of care and concern I received. The hospital's Crisis Team talked with me on several occasions.

I was discharged a few days later under Jack's supervision, and with the name of the mental health nurse who would initiate contact with me once I arrived back in Dannevirke. The Salvation Army arranged for Jack and me to have a week at their downtown Railton hotel, so the hospital had also given us a contact number for support during our remaining time in Auckland.

Whenever I thought about the disgusting, degrading, humiliating experience at the hospital, I felt even more alone in my misery. I vowed that this would never happen to me again.

The next time I will do it right!

2024 Looking Back:
I never had suicidal thoughts in my childhood or adolescence or early adulthood. Now, after long spiritual experience, I better see how much Satan influenced my thought processes with the anorexia. In my early years I was caught completely off guard by the Adversary. He poured his evil ideas and images into my mind, causing me to hate myself. There was little awareness or resistance on my part. *At the same time*, the anorexia was also my armor - *my anorexia armor* - to protect myself from the domestic abuse I was experiencing. Therefore, I was in a spiritual battle where **the anorexia was both *my protection* and *the weapon* I used against myself!** This was because **Jack and Satan had BOTH hijacked me!**

2024 Spiritual Awakening:
We may sometimes attribute our thoughts that feel foreign or evil, to our subconscious mind. That is, they may be a result of our own experiences, emotions, and memories. Yet they may also be influenced by external factors, such as our environment, relationships, and even demonic influences.

Yehovah is the only One who truly knows our thoughts. Satan and his demons do not have the ability to read our minds, but they are opportunists, making educated guesses about our thoughts, and then seeking to tempt and influence our thought processes with their schemes, temptations and deceptions. Satan is clever and logically subtle, mixing both truths and half-truths together with his lies.

Ephesians 6:16 *"Above all, taking the shield of faith with which you will be able to quench all the fiery darts of the wicked one."* Paul speaks of the flaming darts sent by the wicked one (Satan). So how do we recognize fiery darts? Examine the effect the "suspicious thought" has on you. Does it produce fear, doubt, jealousy, inferiority, confusion, judgement, anger, inferiority, selfishness, or a gross misperception of what your body looks like, for example?

In my anorexic thinking and suicidal ideation, I did not understand that I was being bombarded by Satan's fiery darts. I was not wearing my spiritual armor or using my spiritual weapons as I could have been.

What to Do with Fiery Darts

1. **Recognize:** When we experience unwanted thoughts, we must recognize them for what they are – not necessarily a reflection of our true selves, but rather our own subconscious mind, or a result of external influences.

2. **Resist:** Scripture commands us to submit to Yehovah and resist the devil. This means acknowledging that these thoughts are not from Yehovah and choose to reject them. James 4:7-8 has the promise that if we submit to Yehovah and resist the devil, that he will flee from us.

If we are not focused on Yehovah and His truth as we ought to be, daily renewing our minds (Romans 12:1-2), putting on the armor and picking up the weaponry of Yehovah to fight the good fight of faith (Ephesians 6), pleading the blood of Yeshua over our lives, and we fail to respond to Yehovah's grace, we open ourselves up to greater and greater control by Satan. The greater that influence, the more likely he will control our thinking processes and consequent behaviors.

The truth is that Yeshua gave all believers power and authority over every spirit of darkness - especially Satan! If anyone reading this is dealing with anorexia, or has a loved one dealing with anorexia, know that this is a spiritual battle. Take authority over Satan, stand in faith and pray for deliverance. If you do not have the faith yourself, go to someone who does!

CHAPTER 3

I Have Heard Their Cry

...the children of Israel groaned
because of the bondage, and they cried out;
and their cry came up to God because of the bondage.
Exodus 2:23

I was grateful to be staying at the Railton Hotel. At least I was out of the hospital. Jack and I sat in the darkness on the balcony one night. As I viewed the big, colorful and busy city of Auckland, I shared with Jack that I was frightened by the unsafe feelings I had - that it would be so easy to make another attempt at ending my life even in these conducive surrounds. It was a prescient confession. Jack decided I would make no more outings without someone accompanying me.

The bondage of my illness pursued me. Food continued to be a huge issue. It was even harder when I could not plan and prepare what I ate. My mood remained low. I had no ability to just 'live' like everyone else. I still wanted to die, but there was now adequate support holding me upright lest I fall. I was scared to return home. I felt I could easily fall again.

Saturday 16 November 1991
I am desperately unhappy. Life is too hard. I am too fat. It is another day to cope with and struggle through. The desire to exercise constantly and burn calories persists. I do not want to do or be anything. Too little food and too much exercise leaves me with no energy, yet my brain still screams out at me for eating anything! This morning, I got up at 5:00 am. Having told Jack that I was only going to sit on the patio, I snuck out a fire escape door to go for a walk. My movements however were not as discreet as I had planned, as in opening the door I set off the building alarm, before escaping into the darkness undiscovered!

Jack is in discussion with The Salvation Army leaders to decide what needs to happen between now and our upcoming change of appointment. A change of appointment is a regular feature in The Salvation Army, but my mental health crisis precipitates an earlier move. They agreed that a move out of Dannevirke to a more helpful place needs to happen before January. I cannot understand why we are being helped and supported so much.

Sunday 17 November 1991
We left Auckland, to return home, early this morning. The journey from Auckland which passed through Tauranga was almost enjoyable for me. The day was sunny, pleasantly warm, and even… well, beautiful. In contrast to this, Jack and I engaged in a deep and intense conversation about death, dying, suicide and its consequences. He told me how great his pain would be if I killed myself.

2024 Looking Back:
Jack always knew just what to say but he did not always mean it. This expression of "great pain" caused me to believe that he loved me, and that we had a mutually loving relationship. As the years went on his affirmation changed to, *"You'd never make it without me!"* At the time I was unable to recognize Jack's influence on my illness. So I took all the blame on myself, and I hated myself for it. Although Jack always knew the right words to say, I eventually came to see through them. His insincerity was clear in what followed.

*****

We reached Napier early evening on the way back to Dannevirke. After much inner wrangling and discussion with Jack, I made a surprising and decisive decision to have a meat pie and fries for dinner. What a mistake, but then I knew it would be. As soon as I began to eat these forbidden foods I had suddenly craved, I knew I would have to get rid of them from my stomach! I ignored Jack's advice to stop eating. I could have better managed a smaller portion. My mind was telling me that I had already passed the point of no return, and so I compulsively kept stuffing the pie and fries into my mouth.

Immediately after I had finished eating, I begged Jack to take me to a toilet. Jack angrily responded that he would not drive me to McDonald's where I knew the toilets would be clean. He told me I should not have that privilege, and that if I wanted to spew, I should use the town amenities which we knew from prior experience to be filthy and smelly. He stood outside as I began the difficult and disgusting task of reversing. It was hard to bring it up as I stuck my fingers down my throat. It was shameful enough throwing up in your own clean toilet, but to use a dirty public toilet really highlighted the depths of degradation I had sunk to. I made my downcast exit with a raw throat, and a red and swollen face. I was ashamed and in tears as I got back into the car with Jack. I had been punished.

Within the first several days of being back in Dannevirke, the old obsessive and compulsive routines flourished. However, the almost daily visits of a mental health nurse, and the goal of making Christmas cards and gifts that I feverishly embarked on, provided some distraction and relief from my torment and despair.

Our Salvation Army superiors were aware of my mental condition and so gave Jack a new appointment in the finance department at Territorial Headquarters in Wellington. Jack and I would move to Wellington where I could access the outpatient mental health treatment.

Tuesday 26 November 1991

Patricia came through to see me this morning. I found her visit difficult at first, until we started to talk through our recent relationship difficulties. We shared honestly. It helped me greatly to understand that Patricia's responses were her attempts at letting go. She realized that Jack and I would need to be moved away from Dannevirke, and this wasn't easy for her. Patricia told me that her hardness and indifference to me, was in fact her bad attempt at letting me go. She had even been to talk this through with Dr. Andy. Patricia asked me to forgive her, and I did.

Within the week of our return to Dannevirke, our belongings were packed up. As well as this, alternative leadership was found for a month of Sunday services, and various activities and programs were postponed or canceled. The community work skills program had to be left unattended until new Corps officers were appointed to the Dannevirke Corps.

Jack and I then temporarily relocated to the Training College grounds of Upper Hutt, while we waited for The Salvation Army to find us a house in Wellington to live in. From Upper Hutt, Jack made many trips back to Dannevirke until all the responsibilities could be passed on to others. Everyone hoped the familiar surroundings of the Training College would give me more help and support.

Friday 29 November 1991
This eating conflict makes life unbearable. And how can people say *"there is nothing of you"* when I have so much fat! They are either deceived or they are trying to deceive me! I hate my body. It is undisciplined and fat. Today my body once again is worn out from bingeing and purging. Why, why, why, do I do it?

2024 Looking Back:
I look back and see the anguish of my spirit and the cruel bondage of the depression and anorexia. I was crying out to Yehovah just as the children of Israel had cried out to Him, when they were in bondage and slavery in Egypt. Just like them, I could not see my deliverance coming from Yehovah, yet it would come!

*****

2024 Spiritual Awakening:
In Exodus 6, Yehovah speaks to Moses and tells him what He will do for captive Israel. Yehovah says to Moses seven times, *"I will"* regarding how He will save His people!

Yehovah is my covenant-keeping God too. He is the God of the *'I Will'*. He is the God of miracles, signs and wonders. Just as Yehovah brought Israel out of their hopelessness, despair, frustration, fear and depression, He would also deliver me. These are promises *we can all* bank on!

Then Yehovah said to Moses,

*"Now you shall see what **I will** do to Pharaoh..."*

And God spoke to Moses and said to him: "I am Yehovah.
I appeared to Abraham, to Isaac, and to Jacob, as El Shaddai,

but by My name Yehovah I was not known to them.
I have also established My covenant with them,
to give them the land of Canaan, the land of their pilgrimage,
in which they were strangers.

And I have also heard the groaning of the children of Israel whom the Egyptians keep in bondage,
and I have remembered My covenant.
Therefore say to the children of Israel: 'I am Yehovah;

***I will** bring you out from under the burdens of the Egyptians,*
***I will** rescue you from their bondage, and*
***I will** redeem you with an outstretched arm*
and with great judgments.

***I will** take you as My people, and **I will** be your God.*
Then you shall know that I am Yehovah your God who brings you out from under the burdens of the Egyptians.

*And **I will** bring you into the land which I swore*
to give to Abraham, Isaac, and Jacob; and

***I will** give it to you as a heritage: I am Yehovah.' "*

So Moses spoke thus to the children of Israel; but they did not heed Moses, because of anguish of spirit and cruel bondage.

Exodus 6 :1-9

*****

Sunday 8 December 1991

Having Rebekah and Richard at the Training College is the best thing about being here again. It seems strange to return to the place that was the catalyst for my destruction. Now, I have no responsibilities and there are no expectations of me. I frequently walk with Rebekah in the evenings. It's a good opportunity for us to talk.

Monday 9 December 1991

I don't feel good about seeing this new doctor at Wellington Hospital. I now have to start all over again with someone unfamiliar. I am told that treating anorexics is her thing. Huh! I am a fraud. I have recently been eating so much and am so fat. Dr. Hill will take one look at me and wonder why I am there!

Tuesday 17 December 1991

My mind continues to be an evil den of inner confusion, conflict and torment. The other night I went for an accompanied walk with Valorie, another Salvation Army officer on staff at the College. Valorie made a number of unsuccessful attempts to initiate conversation as we walked along by the Hutt River. She told me the next day that she decided to give up. These 'destroyers of my mind,' so assaulting and intense, made it impossible for me to voice even the smallest utterance, and so we walked in silence for most of that one and a half hours. As we crossed the Hutt motorway, I had tears pouring down my face as I thought of how easily I could step in front of one of those cars and end it all.

Saturday 21 December 1991

Today we moved into the Wellington suburb of Kingston, where Jack and I will now live. It's a tidy two-bedroom duplex apartment on the top of a hill near the end of a cul-de-sac. We have a view of the Cook Strait, a private sun-bathing spot, a good crop of mint, orange carpet in the bedrooms and a letter box that refuses to open! Besides these features, the wind is buffeting the house from every direction.

*****

Moving house again was exhausting, but I was grateful for the relief this relocation offered. No longer was I prisoner in my own home as I had felt in Dannevirke, and the location gave me plenty of challenging walking opportunities to complement my daily Exercycle regime. I had a new and greater selection of pharmacies to oblige my addiction to laxatives.

Within the Wellington area were a great many kind and caring people I knew, who were ready with offers of help, support and friendship. Despite this, I believed few had the capacity to adequately understand my situation and support me. So, I was reluctant to reach out.

Ana, a Salvation Army officer colleague who lived in Wellington, was one person who I did allow to help and support me when circumstances forced my hand. It was time with Ana, and telephone calls to Rebekah in Upper Hutt, that continued to be vital for me. Our contact with Patricia and Ed had become less regular.

The type of relationships I had previously had with people before I became unwell, changed. What were once comfortable and relaxed relationships, had become formal and correct. On their part there was uncertainty, and fear of saying or doing the wrong thing - and ignorance. On my part, I kept people at a distance due to my fears and eating disorder obsessions.

The finance department of The Salvation Army Territorial Headquarters was Jack's new appointment. He was in a training role that allowed him a measure of flexibility to accommodate our circumstances.

*****

Tuesday 31 December 1991
It is the last day of a long, dark and unhappy year. I can’t go through another twelve months like these.

Saturday 11 January 1992
The first days of this year have generally been better. I have laughed and joked, which has not happened in months.

Since moving to Wellington, I've felt like I have been held together by more positive circumstances, but I don't know if they will last. Jack starts work on Monday. I'm looking forward to some independence and freedom, but I'm also scared that my eating will go crazy again. While Jack has been with me and managing my eating with me, it has been more normal - not that I feel okay about that. I am taking more laxatives than he knows.

I weigh 53 kilograms (116 lbs). I feel like 10 tons!

Sunday 12 January 1992
The tormenting conflict between my obsession and denial continually threaten to overwhelm me. Yesterday afternoon, I got into the pasta, baked beans and cheese. Then a cake. Of course, the final phase of 'reversing' followed. If only I could believe it was okay for me to eat a piece of cake, then maybe I would not be compelled to gorge on it all before getting rid of it all. Every time I 'reverse' it feels like I was losing a battle in the war. The disappointment and shame is intense.

Monday 13 January 1992
On this wet and miserable afternoon, I had my first appointment with Dr. Ann Hill at Wellington Hospital's Psychiatric Out-Patient's Department. I was scared to go, and sitting in the waiting area was creepy. All I wanted to do was escape from that ugly and run-down mental place!

Dr. Hill was like an old school mistress. I had to endure an intimidating two and a half hours with her, while aware that a Registrar was viewing me from behind a two-way mirror. I was to have seen Dr. Hill alone, but once her barrage of questions started, I left the room and dragged Jack in. It was more than I could cope with, alone. I was relieved that Jack then did most of the talking for me. When more straight forward questions were directed at me, I could not answer these honestly as Jack had little or no awareness of my secretive behavior.

Dr. Hill's manner upset me. Surely she could have gotten the same information in a nicer way! Apparently she was going to whip me into shape! I left Dr. Hill's office in a tearful and worn-out state. I want Dr. Andy back!

Wednesday 15 January 1992

I am still unhappy and low. I feel shame in the eyes of friends and The Salvation Army leaders. I also feel shame when I hear people making insensitive and ignorant comments about eating disorders and sufferers. They seem disgusted with us.

Jack and I walked the Kingston and Brooklyn hills tonight. We talked about how I have always hated what is inside me, and therefore have hidden my real self from others for fear of them seeing and hating it too. He likened it to me only letting people see the shop front but giving them no permission to enter.

2024 Looking Back:

I realize that I never hated myself when I was younger nor was I hiding who I was. The nature of Jack's controlling relationship with me and Satan's fiery darts, conditioned me to believe this. Then, once my subconscious accepted it, these messages became engrained in my mind.

Thursday 16 January 1992

I have again accumulated enough money for my 'illegal' laxatives - these are the additional ones that no one knows I am taking. Under the pretense of needing a bus fare into town, Jack will give me money. Unbeknownst to Jack, I have never been on a bus into town! Why would I be so lazy when I can walk the hills and get rid of some fat?

I acquire laxatives without money sometimes. I've become good at this. The other day I even shoplifted a packet of pearl beads. I didn't go to the shop with this intention, and I didn't need or want them. Perhaps I was testing God.

I lie, I steal, I abuse my body,
I hurt and destroy others…
Do you still love me now Mister God?

2024 Looking Back:
This question I wrote in my journal, came out of my shame and self condemnation. I desperately wanted to know that He still loved me, but I could not see how He could. 'Mister God' surely did still love me, but I had allowed Satan's megaphone voice to tell me otherwise.

But You, Yehovah, are a God full of compassion, and gracious, long-suffering and abundant in mercy and truth.
Psalm 86:15

*****

Thursday 16 January 1992 (continued)
My 'look-alike' African violet plant that made the move with us to Wellington has some new growth on it. This house provides better conditions for it. The new growth is forming lop-sided though, and looks weird. There are still no flowers.

My spiritual state now is extremely different from the past. I had always been seen as spiritual by others. I had believed this myself. Now there is nothing of that in me. I do not have, and I cannot be, anything spiritual. My spiritual image is smashed. I now have no image to maintain and nothing to lose.

God, can't you talk to me? What am I to do?

2024 Spiritual Awakening:
My mind was like a radio, and instead of it being tuned to the truth of Yehovah's Word, I had it tuned to the lies of the Cruel Master, Satan's radio station. I was letting the words of untruth "*dwell in me*" with the volume turned up loud!

I had a very clear reception of the Cruel Master's station, but the true voice station of Yehovah's Word was almost impossible to pick up. It faded in and out, and I got a lot of interference.

To overcome anorexia, I would have to want Yehovah's true voice station, "*dwell in me richly*," to once again hear my loving Heavenly Father speaking to me.

Let the word of Messiah dwell in you richly,
teaching and admonishing one another in all wisdom,
singing psalms and hymns and spiritual songs,
with thankfulness in your hearts to God.
Colossians 3:16

Friday 17 January 1992
Over recent days I have again been overwhelmed and unable to cope or do the simplest things. Jack has had to literally lift me up from where I'm sitting. I'm angry with life and ungrateful for it. It's too hard. I wish I had a choice about living, instead of it being imposed upon me!

Sunday 26 January 1992
Eating is such a complicated business. Everything I eat creates the great problem of how to overcome the consequences. 5:30 am is my start time of the day. I get my exercise done before Jack gets up. I am still not sleeping well.

I saw the dentist this week with my referral letter from Dr. Hill. I felt ashamed as the dentist read of my anorexia and probable dental problems. Thankfully, he was sensitive to my feelings.

Sunday 2 February 1992
My birthday on Monday was a bad day. Mum and Dad came to visit me while Jack was at work. I was left feeling hurt because my mother did not say anything significant or meaningful. Sure, she said *"I love you,"* but this means little to me when it is meant to substantiate everything else unspoken.

I had an appointment with the hospital dietitian during the week. She is meant to help me view food in a more balanced way.

2024 Looking Back:
The anorexia created a huge abyss between us. My parents were the bad guys in this therapy scenario which encouraged me to think my problems began in childhood. It had warped my attitudes towards my parents. Now, the simple expression, "I love you" came to mean very little to me. My parents, particularly my mother, did not give any acknowledgment of my being unwell, and so I felt forced into a place of having to appear well and coping while in their presence. The truth was, they were having to walk on eggshells around me, not knowing what to say or do.

Tuesday 4 February 1992
The days are so long. I am not coping well with life. I am bingeing regularly again. I hate admitting this failure. Often, I am not honest when Jack asks me of any eating plans before he goes to work - especially if it has been planned since the previous night and I am intent on carrying it through. There is no hope for me once I reach the point of no return and start bingeing yet again.

Tuesday 11 February 1992
Life is too hard and without purpose and pleasure. I am so unhappy. Yesterday and today, I am feeling so distant. I continue to wonder how situations would be without me around. I have little motivation and energy for anything. I don't think my life will ever be of value. I want to die.

I cannot tell others how desperate I feel. To give the same sad story makes me feel like a pathetic attention seeker. I keep remembering Frank and Milly's words - that what I was saying to them about not wanting to live was a load of crap! They were wrong. And now, why would I give others the opportunity to think or say the same thing?

It is best not to say anything at all to anyone!

Thursday 13 February 1992
I went to Palmerston North to see Dr. Andy today. It was a comfort visit for me. Finally I could talk and be with someone who knew and understood me. It has been a long time. I felt hopeless though with Andy too. Surely he must be sick of the sight of me, although he said he wasn't.

Last week the dietitian told me that I am the first patient in her career, where she is at a loss as to how to help. Great! She has validated my feelings of hopelessness. Then my appointment with Dr. Hill followed… I still didn't appreciate her brisk manner, but this time she communicated some care and concern. She was even sorry for her three weeks absence. As well as prescribing anti-depressants for me, she asked if an admission to the hospital would be a helpful option.

Well… I have had no intention of taking the medication. At least not as prescribed! How stupid was she to put so many tablets in my hands! And no, the psychiatric unit has no appeal to me - perhaps the morgue does!

Tuesday 18 February 1992
I feel like a freak. People visit and talk all around the subject of me. They don't relate in the slightest on a personal level. Do they fear I will 'crack'? Even those supposedly trained to care for people must think I'll fall apart. I think this myself often enough.

We received a pastoral visit today and were talked to about the weather, the garden, and the church program. Within the one hour that seemed more like ten, we weren't even asked how we were or how things were going! Why is it so hard for most people to be anything other than superficial?

I'm messed up. Jack has decided to just work half days again to babysit me! Our fourth wedding anniversary has been and gone. It seems more like 24 years!

It seems so simple to others just to stick with an eating plan. It only works to the extent that I am honest. My food thoughts rage untamed, and my fears of increased weight seem ridiculous to others. They can't see an increase of my weight, in spite of my increased consumption. That's because I am having to increase my exercise and laxatives. I am desperate to see Dr. Andy. My world is a vicious cycle that is wearing me out. I got my prescription of sleeping tablets today.

She is loyal and doesn't want to betray her abuser.
It's difficult for her to realize how his actions are wrong,
much less abusive, even though she knows how
much pain they cause her. This especially makes it
difficult for her to reach out for help.
Natalie Hoffman - Is It Me?

Wednesday 19 February 1992
I have been extremely low last night and this morning. I have no interest in life. It is a pointless effort. I talked with Rebekah on the phone last night, although she had to do all the talking. I felt disassociated. I was too afraid to share my innermost thoughts and feelings. This morning I suffered a 'near death experience' having over-dosed on laxatives last night. I knew I took too many but I just didn't care. The worst of it began to hit once Jack had left for work. Hours of profuse sweating, diarrhea and stomach cramps.

Friday 21 February 1992
We drove out to Upper Hutt for me to talk with Rebekah. If I was to be honest with anyone about what was going on inside me, it would be her. But not today. Rebekah was expecting us and had dressed ready for the great out-doors that the two of us frequently shared together. After Rebekah had offered her opening remarks in the hope of encouraging a verbal out-pour, we embarked on our usual marathon walk in an uncharacteristic silence. Having said that she would say nothing until I had invited her to, she couldn't resist after forty minutes of uneasy silence.

It didn't take much perception, a gift Rebekah has plenty of, for her to sense my deep despondency and despair. The usual soul-style communion we shared had been drowned by the raging torrent of my resistance and indifference. I was determined to remain closed and isolated as I incurred Rebekah's onslaught of clever crisis counselling skill and her passionate personal concern for me.

In the middle of the golf course where we'd had many fine conversations, Rebekah stopped. My only intention with this walk was to get it over and done with as quickly as possible without any 'spillages.' Rebekah seemed to deliberately slow down our usual pace and had now stopped. I carried on walking until I was thwarted by guilt. I did not want to have to see Rebekah's crippled countenance, so I stood at a distance with my back turned. I tried to convey my readiness to move on as I idly kicked the fallen leaves and stared into the twilight images that this expansive, serene and secluded area presently possessed.

I was not going to make it easy for her to penetrate my resolve. Rebekah had to come to me if there was to be any hope of communication. Her move towards me was deliberate but slow. I responded to her imploring touch by telling her that I had nothing to say. Of course by now she had realized my sense of hopelessness and unspoken intentions of death.

She requested we sit on a nearby seat. I unwillingly agreed. It was only the tears and obvious distress of Rebekah that created a crack in my resistance. She was a dear and loved friend who had given much of her time and self to me in the recent months. I really didn't think I meant even half as much to her as she had meant to me, and so I was puzzled as to why she should be displaying such grief.

In the most rational manner I could, I told Rebekah that I had made an unchangeable decision - no more was I going to cause anyone else pain and hurt. Even the obvious pain of the moment that my life was causing her, further validated my judgement.

My final words to Rebekah, who I knew to be stringently true to her ethics and integrity, was to vow her to secrecy. I told her that I would not forgive her if she broke this confidence. I didn't realize at the time that for her to carry the sole responsibility of this knowledge only served to heighten her pain and grief.

By this stage I told her that I was going whether she walked with me or not. The silence was reinstated until we neared the Training College when Rebekah said in an emotionally broken voice that she must share my words with Laurence - that for her to bear them alone was too much. I could not look into her eyes, as she had wanted me to, when she said this. It would have further threatened to crack my hard exterior. Whatever words Rebekah spoke to me that evening quickly dissipated. Rebekah called Jack the next day in an attempt to express her deep concern for me without breaking her vow of confidentiality.

Adults with a history of having an eating disorder
are nearly 5-6 times more likely to attempt suicide
compared to those who have never had an eating disorder.
Suicide is the leading cause of death for
those with anorexia nervosa.
Udo, T., Bitley, S., & Grilo, C. M. (2019)
Suicide attempts in US adults with DSM-5 eating disorders.
BCM Medicine

Saturday 22 February 1992

I have no energy for living. I have lost all interest in life. The inner conflicts with food are no longer overwhelming and controlling my mind. I have decided to end my life on Monday when no one is around. I am now preoccupied with Monday and how I will communicate the reasons for my actions.

I feel lonely and isolated, but I do not want to share or talk with anyone. There is concern about my apparent lack of openness with anyone. At the beginning of the week I thought I would burst if I could not let out all the reasons for my guilt. I desperately wanted to talk with someone. However, since then things have changed. I am walking a tight-rope. I do not want anyone to know my inner-most feelings, thoughts and plans. I do not want anyone to stop me!

All attempts to work out what is going on inside of me are failing because I am covering it up. This only adds further to my guilt.

I am tired, but my reason for staying in bed longer the last few mornings and returning to bed in the afternoon is to pass the day away. Waiting for Monday seems endless. Every hour is an eternity.

Sunday 23 February 1992
I cannot know for sure that this attempt will be successful. Part of me would want it to succeed, while another part does not. I want to die but I do not want to kill myself. But I have no choice now. My resolve is certain.

God could save me, I suppose.
This will test Him.
I cannot imagine though that my life would mean anything to Him.

The weather was an accurate reflection of my mood when I woke on Monday morning. It was a still grey day. Over recent months I had felt continual grayness within me. However today, the usual accompanying inner turmoil had been stilled as I anticipated a resolution and escape.

I knew that if I failed to answer one of Jack's check-up calls, he would immediately come home. Monday was one of his two mornings a week at Wellington Polytechnic. Therefore, I knew I had a little over two hours before he would make his first routine check-up call.

So today was the most opportune time to execute my well-conceived plans. Any pain I did feel was for myself. I loved Jack and did not want to be without him, yet it was a price I was willing to pay. For Jack there would finally be freedom and relief from the past twelve months of hell I had put him through.

Many (eating disorder) patients reach a point
where they feel they simply can't do it anymore.
Whether it's that they're physically exhausted from the
complications of the disease or they're mentally exhausted,
they reach a stage of giving up.
For many, these feelings are also coupled with the
burden they feel they've placed on their families.
Connie Quinn, DSW, LCSW-R,
Director: The Renfrew Center of New York

2024 Looking Back:
Jack wanted to control me, and he lost control. He wanted me sick and dependent, not suicidal and hospitalized. He was in over his head and had no idea how to reign in the seriousness of the situation. He did the only thing he knew to do, which was to keep exerting power and control over me. I would get better for a time through faith, therapy and sheer determination, then he would pull me back to a place of dependent un-wellness. He did not intend for me to die. I felt unworthy of him, deserving only to die.

2024 Spiritual Awakening:
Satan is a liar. He had me convinced that I could not continue fighting this spiritual battle, that I was not worth this life I had been given! Giving up can seem easier than waiting for Yehovah to save us.

I know the Israelites lost heart in the wilderness and began wanting to die rather than trusting Yehovah. *"If only we had died by Yehovah's hand in Egypt"* was their lament (Exodus 16:3). Yet they had their covenant-keeping God - the 'I will' God - who had proved Himself many times over that He was well able to care for their needs and deliver them. Yehovah was the God of mighty wonders and miracles! And still is! It surprises us that they were not believing or expecting for this, but Yehovah keeps His Word, and He never leaves or forsakes His children. Ever.

And I had this same covenant-keeping God who was going to get me through this time of distress, even while I was like the Israelites wanting to die and not believe or trust God with Whom nothing is impossible, El-Shaddai - God Almighty!

As with the Israelites in Egypt and then in the wilderness, our Abba-Yehovah always hears our cries for help. Even while I was emotionally and spiritually wounded, all I had needed to do was call on The Name of Yehovah to be saved.

Whoever calls on The Name of Yehovah shall be saved.
Romans 10:13

Just as quitting is never an option for a trained soldier in combat, even if wounded, it is not an option for the man or woman of Yehovah to quit. We must stand on His Word as a soldier in His army.

I love Yehovah, because He has heard
My voice and my supplications.

Because He has inclined His ear to me,
Therefore I will call upon Him as long as I live.

The pains of death surrounded me,
And the pangs of Sheol laid hold of me;
I found trouble and sorrow.

Then I called upon The Name of Yehovah:
"O Yehovah I implore You, deliver my soul!"

Gracious is Yehovah, and righteous; Yes, our God is merciful.

Yehovah preserves the simple; I was brought low, and He saved me.

Return to your rest, O my soul,
For Yehovah has dealt bountifully with you.

For You have delivered my soul from death,
My eyes from tears, And my feet from falling.

I will walk before Yehovah in the land of the living.
Psalm 116:1-9

We are called to battle and are destined to win, if we do not give up. However, we are not going to fight a spiritual battle with natural ability and strength, because it is not enough. But, if we fight a spiritual battle with Yehovah's power, authority and dominion, as recorded in Luke 10:19, we will win. Even if we are spiritually or emotionally compromised or 'wounded' - e.g. oppressed, depressed, suicidal, despairing, fearful - we are to call on the name of Yehovah, and we shall be saved. We can still fight the enemy while afflicted.

We must believe that Yehovah's Word is true when it claims that He will come through for us as long as we do not give up. Back then, I was not standing on the Word of Yehovah for my deliverance. I lost heart many times.

Whatever difficulty we are facing, now or in these days ahead, we must stand on the powerful truth of Yehovah's Word until victory is achieved. As end-time saints, this is especially important for us. We must not give up. Ever. We must put on the full armor that Yehovah has given us (see Ephesians 6:13-20).

*****

As soon as Jack had shut the door behind him, I was out of bed with an uncharacteristic burst of energy. The need to have my house in perfect order was a priority, so the dishes were done, the bed made, and the few things lying around were put away. I then got myself showered and dressed. It seemed wrong to leave a mess behind, or to look a mess myself.

Of all the options I had considered, over-dosing on medication was the least messy way to end my life. I knew that the 180 antidepressant tablets combined with the 10 sleeping tablets were more than sufficient. I then taped a letter to Jack on the inside of the front door.

Jack,

My life has somehow become a web of vicious downward cycles, and this has made it increasingly difficult for me to be honest with you about so many things.

Because of this I feel much guilt... Well the truth is I am guilty! I cannot cope with feeling like this any longer. It really is just too much for me to bear... This is an expression of cowardice, and a punishment for my guilt.

Please forgive me.

Cate

Already experiencing the effects of the first handful of tablets, I took the remaining dishful and curled up. I had an awareness of my surroundings for only a short time. The sentence had been passed. The judgement had been carried out.

A HARD DAY'S NIGHT

Jack had driven to the Poly-Technical Institute that morning. When he returned home he was greeted by my note. Finding me in an unconscious and trembling state, he rang 111, New Zealand's emergency number. He looked around the house for tablet boxes, and once he had assessed the situation as best he could, he made telephone calls to inform Rebekah, his mother and his work while waiting for the sound of an ambulance siren.

The attendants' attempts at trying to arouse me proved unsuccessful. Oxygen was administered, and within a short space of time I had been maneuvered onto a stretcher, hustled down the steps into the ambulance and taken to Wellington's Public Hospital.

Jack later told me that he had told God not to bother letting me live if the eating disorder and depression cycle was to continue! He was well aware of the implications of my actions having been put through this situation only months before. The senselessness of what I had done fueled his anger. He was no longer in control. I was taking back control in the only way I knew how.

The hospital orderlies took me into the Accident and Emergency department. The admitting office staff wanted Jack to fill in forms. The perfunctory manner in which they carried out their routine work expressed no recognition of the significance of the situation. As a team of about six doctors and nurses began working on me, they were ushered into a small office. Jack was told they would fetch him if there was likelihood of my death.

As friends began arriving Jack felt forced to maintain his ever-present characteristic strength, presence of mind, and protection for a now helpless and speechless Cate. The group congregated in the waiting area as if awaiting a verdict. They were told that there was doubt as to whether I would survive. If I did live, I would possibly sustain brain damage and, or, my heart could fail because of its inability to cope with the full effect of the overdose. They pumped my stomach, but too much had already been absorbed into my system. There was no antidote.

They had to wait for the full effect to peak before knowing the consequences. I was transferred to the Intensive Care Unit. I lay wrapped in a tin foil blanket to minimize the hypothermia, with an airway pipe, oxygen, and tube up through my nose. I was a picture of pathos.

My parents were contacted and told I might not make it. Other family members were notified. As I lay unconscious, various people visited me through the afternoon and evening. It was all too much for some to see me like this. My sister-in-law was one who spent only a brief time with me before leaving in tears.

My parents arrived in Wellington late evening. They had wanted to be the ones to stay with me throughout the night hours. Jack communicated to them that it would have been the most unhelpful thing for me, especially if I were to regain consciousness and find them at my bedside. He was only willing to leave me in Rebekah's care once my parents had been required to leave for the night. By this time it was around midnight.

2024 Looking Back:
It might seem odd to the reader that my parents were not wanted in the hospital room of their daughter who was on the verge of dying. Remember that all of the blame for my anorexia, depression and suicidal behavior had been laid on the doorstep of my parents. My parents had been cast as the villains of this life-threatening physical and mental illness. Jack said it. I believed it. Everyone else, from doctors to nurses to therapists to friends, agreed with it. It is an enduring heartbreak to me, that my loving parents were saddled with such guilt and shame by me and so many others. It took a lot longer for me to realize that Jack was the driver of this disease.

*****

Yeshua calls His own by name and leads them

But now, thus says Yehovah, who created you, O Jacob,
And He who formed you, O Israel:
"Fear not, for I have redeemed you;
I have called *<u>you</u>* *by your* ***name;***
You *<u>are</u>* ***Mine.****"*
Isaiah 43:1

Rebekah spent the night hours praying, talking and singing to me. I remember the dark stillness as I regained consciousness. The silence was broken only by Rebekah singing to me the words of a song I knew "*..for His love remains the same, He knows you by your name. Don't think, because you've failed Him, He despairs....*" I made no response to her immediately as I lay trying to work things out in my mind. I could not think beyond the realization that I was alive. I was in hospital. God had not let me die. Rebekah's very presence was expressing yet more of her love for me. Why, after it had been so horrible for her the last time we walked together, leaving her heartbroken and in tears?

When Rebekah became aware of my consciousness, she told me who she was, and where I was. All I could say to her was, *"You must be tired Rebekah."*

I merely existed through the hours that followed. Jack came. Rebekah went. Medical staff pulled and poked at me. Visitors came who said little but were obviously attempting to convey much. What was to become of me now? Surely I was just a nuisance to the nurses and doctors. Though Jack was being considerate of me, I was not receiving any overt or convincing expressions that he was pleased I was still alive.

For I know the thoughts that I think toward you, says Yehovah, thoughts of peace and not of evil, to give you a future and a hope.
Jeremiah 29:11

*****

2024 Spiritual Awakening:
Yehovah is all about loving relationships - husbands and wives, parents and children, brothers and sisters. Yehovah models, and even participates, in these relationships with us! We have the children of Israel entering into a marriage covenant with Him at Mt. Sinai. In the household of faith, of those keeping the Torah of Yehovah (see Mark 3:35), we are brothers and sisters. Yeshua is also our brother.

Marriage is important to Yehovah. My mother and father had demonstrated to me a loving husband and wife relationship. I entered into a marriage that was something other than love.

In the Bible account of Hosea and Gomer (see Hosea):

Gomer kept getting drawn down into darkness. She chose it, but like us, regardless of how we get into the darkness, we are confused. Our thinking can be jumbled, even the things we know to be real, true and right. It is in the persistent love of the Groom Yeshua - who comes back for us and says, *"I am trustworthy, I love you. It doesn't matter where you've been and what you've done"* - that we can become whole and holy and have our vision clear. However, we can be continually drawn to that darkness, because it is familiar. This might be why many women choose the same type of husband, over and over, who will abuse them. They are deceived into thinking that it is like 'home' - a place they know.

The Israelites had the love of Yehovah, but they kept turning away and becoming unfaithful. Then in their distress they would cry out to Yehovah and He would rescue them. Every time. Still, they would inevitably revert back to their pagan and idolatrous ways. Even when the children of Israel were faithless, Yehovah remained faithful - He remained a faithful husband to Israel. Yeshua remains the faithful groom to His bride - believers in Messiah.

Thursday 27 February 1992
I am still here. I have failed a second attempt to end my life. I cannot even get this simple thing right! I am angry about my predicament. Life continues to be imposed upon me.

Friday 28 February 1992
I was transferred to a medical ward later in the day. Ed and Patricia and my parents visited me. The shame I felt was mixed with the feeling of nothingness. It seemed to me that I was treated as an outcast by ward staff. Now I am in the psych unit and feel more freakier than ever! I made it quite clear that I did not want to be here and pleaded with the nurse and registrar to let me go home. A psychiatrist came and gave me the choice to either stay here at the Wellington unit or be committed to the Porirua Psychiatric Hospital. So, what sort of choice did I have?

Everything within me is acting like an obstinate and rebellious child. I am not doing what they want me to do. I am not saying what they want me to say. I will not eat what they want me to eat. The first day I cried all day. My first impressions and experiences of this place only added to my inconsolable state. I watched zombie patients dressed in hospital pajamas walking up and down the corridors. All my belongings were checked for dangerous objects and medications. I was told that for the first two days I had to wear hospital pajamas! To this I declared my utmost resistance. Eventually they decided to break hospital policy and allow me to remain in my clothes. This was small comfort for the devastation I felt. I was a mess when Valorie visited in the afternoon.

*****

2024 Looking Back:
As with the events of my first suicide attempt, this chapter was very painful and distressing for me to write and reread. I realized that even after so many years since these events took place, there were toxic emotions from this time that had remained in my soul, bringing me to tears. There were toxic emotions of: shame, failure, depression, hopelessness, despair, embarrassment and humiliation.

Clearly, I needed more healing. In prayer I have now released these toxic emotions to Yeshua and asked Him to heal the wounds these toxic emotions inflicted on my soul. As I received Yeshua's love and forgiveness to heal me, I then saw in my mind a beach scene. I was looking at the darkened wet sand, close to the water's edge. The sand had been greatly disturbed and messed-up. It looked scarred and wounded!

Then came gentle waves of the ocean washing up over this messed up sand. As each incoming wave of the ocean made its way to the shoreline and over the messed up sand, the sand started to level out and smooth. Wave after wave came until there was no remaining evidence of the sand having ever been disturbed. The beach was left looking as it does at the start of a new day before anyone has come - pristine and inviting!

I realized I was being given a picture of Yeshua's love and forgiveness, washing over my scarred and wounded soul. Wave after gentle wave of Yeshua's love and forgiveness cleansing and healing my soul of the wounds these toxic emotions had caused. And then came the verse….

As far as the east is from the west,
so far has He (Yehovah) removed our transgressions from us.
Psalm 103:12

Thank you, Father!

****

Friday 28 February 1992 (continued)
I had not talked with anyone else until Thursday when I met another patient on the ward. As soon as I talked with her, I realized it was a mistake. She was a Christian! Within a short period of time she had given me her complete medical and spiritual history, and told me about every prayer and prophecy she had ever received. She was delighted to have found another Christian. I wasn't. I felt repelled by Christian attitudes and platitudes.

Over the past year I have rejected and separated myself from all outward shows of faith and the associated expectations. It has been too much for me to cope with. God has continued to be far away - unable or unwilling to penetrate the bubble of my existence. Even though God had apparently spared me, I didn't see the point. To have succumbed to this patient's probing questions and tell her I was a Christian, was a bad enough mistake to make, but then to say I was a Salvation Army Officer - I am nuts! I very quickly told her that if she thought I could be a reciprocating help to her, she was wrong. I have not spoken to anyone else since.

One reason for my distress is that I am now on the other side of the fence. I am the patient instead of the nurse. Worse still is the stigma of needing psychiatric help. This is shame and humiliation. Perhaps I too had expressed the same condescending attitudes to psychiatric patients as I am now experiencing.

Sunday 1 March 1992
I hate being in the loony bin. There is little privacy in the showers, and the toilets doors have no locks. Patients are continually checked to ensure they have not escaped! There are no open windows. The door to the ward is locked each night at 8:30 pm.

Monday 2 March 1992
As I lay in my hospital bed last night I was overwhelmed by a spiritual aloneness. I have not felt quite like this before. In my mind, I pictured myself behind a great big fence. Beyond the fence was God and His comfort which I so desperately craved. It was comfort I could only see but have no part of. The intensity of distress this created, led me to ring Ana. Among the words she spoke were, *"nothing can separate us from the love of God"* (see Romans 8:31-39). I had not read or allowed anyone to quote Scripture to me for over a year!

This verse hugely impacted me last night and has brought me to a turning point. Although the desire for death has gone and I feel like a sponge that wants to soak up all available comfort, I do not feel elevated or euphoric. I am not going to pretend a spiritual experience and get myself back into an old rut. I will be true to what I feel and do not feel, and God will have to settle for this honesty.

Coinciding with this very significant happening, the struggling-to-survive African violet plant at home, has a bud I am told! No longer is this African violet barely alive. It too has reached a turning point.

*****

CHAPTER 4

Let There Be Light

There was thick darkness in all the land of Egypt three days...
But all the children of Israel had ***light in their dwellings****.*
Exodus 10:22-23

Do not rejoice over me, my enemy; When I fall, I will arise;
When I sit in darkness, Yehovah will be a light to me.
Micah 7:8

Friday 6 March 1992
Yesterday I was moved from the acute area to a bed at the other end of the ward. I should have been grateful for a more peaceful location, but instead I felt isolated. With this transition I threw out most of the flowers I had been given. These flowers had been visible evidence to me of people's care. I didn't want to wait till the flowers were dead before I threw them out. That would have only served to heighten my feelings of aloneness.

Being in bed through the dark night hours had not been a restful or pleasant experience for a long while. I dread the nighttime which seems an eternity in my sleeplessness. Having some form of light is a measure of comfort, so I've been sleeping with the curtains pulled back to let the moonlight in.

One night in the darkness of the ward and the darkness of my soul, I had a profound experience - a turning point. As I lay in bed in the blackness of the ward listening to music on my Walkman, **a sky-light window shone a shaft of light down on to the floor near my bed! The music and light enveloped me in an overwhelming optimism for life. My life!**

I lay basking in the wonderment of this unfamiliar feeling, and thought I would burst! Was this real? I began to think of all the people I would like to tell of this transformation. Yehovah was giving me the promise of a way out of the darkness, giving me His light to find the way. It embedded a desire in me to live and get better. From now on, my therapy team: Carmia, Chrissy and Caitlin would have my full cooperation!

We may not know how we're going to win the battle, but hold on... Yehovah does!

2024 Spiritual Awakening:

Indeed, the darkness shall not hide from You,
But the night shines as the day;
The darkness and the light are both alike to You.
Psalm 139:12

***Yehovah will fight for you**, and you shall hold your peace.*
Exodus 14:14

Saturday 7 March 1992
Last night Patricia rang me. She seemed skeptical of the change in me until I explained things more fully. She told me that while I was in the hospital, a group of Palmerston North teenagers had been praying that I would receive **'a shaft of light.'** We were both amazed!

Patricia told me that I have been in her prayer journal since the beginning of last year, along with many other requests she had made of God. I was the only unanswered prayer. She could not understand why, and told me that she thought it was the end of me when I overdosed on Monday.

Sunday 8 March 1992
Today I rang our dear friends Rob and Lisa in Christchurch to tell them how different I was feeling. Rob told me that he had been

praying that I would receive **'a shaft of light.'** Ha! This was a second incredible confirmation! I told him that this was *exactly* what had happened to me the other night, and even the same words. God is present and interested in my life.

2024 Looking Back:
I am still moved that the Holy Spirit was giving instruction to others on the way to pray for me. There were people in two different islands of New Zealand praying for the very same thing - that I would receive a **'shaft of light',** and that is exactly what I experienced!

Friday 13 March 1992
Rebekah and Richard visited on Tuesday. One of the things that comes to my mind as I think back to my time at the Training College was a passionate Bible message Laurence gave us from Isaiah. While he was here with me the other day he reminded me of the same key verse.".. *a bruised reed He will not break...*" Isaiah 42:3.

Although optimism is still with me, Wednesday was a low day— as is every day that I am weighed. I have been completely honest, and doing the right things with my eating since the other Sunday, but the staff are still watching me like a hawk.

Today is yet another day when I remember what Dr. Andy once told me. That God is BIG - BIG enough to let me be and do nothing yet still love me. Even BIG enough to love me while doing wrong and destructive things. Only over recent days have I started to believe this, and at those times **when some insight of His love comes, that optimism gushes within me!**

I'm not excusing myself to my visitors anymore for being in a psychiatric ward. I feel like a sponge - nothing to give others but craving and absorbing what comfort others will give me. I have come to see that I'm not the only sane one amongst the insane. I identify with other patients here. One of them is Susan. She is younger than me. We've been talking. She has attempted suicide by over-dosing three times. This is so sad, but I get it.

While Susan and I were at Occupational Therapy the other day we talked together about what we had each over-dosed on. We were like two small children sitting in the playground asking what the other had in their lunchbox. It could have been overheard by someone as a flippant conversation on a matter of life and death. Not so.

The only difference now between Susan and me is that I have some hope. I was open and real with her as I have been with the doctors and my nurses about what and why things have changed and are changing for me. That is, that I know God saved me. I am beginning to realize something of His love for me, and something of His help.

Monday 16 March 1992
I am apprehensive about going home tomorrow. I don't want to fall again. The doctor is telling me that I am bound to have slip-ups and set-backs along the way - to even expect to take two steps forward and one step back. I know that old patterns and behaviors are hard to let go. Even in this supportive and safe environment it has been hard work. I will have plenty of out-patient support, the doctor tells me that being at home will feel as if I am learning to ride a bicycle in the Swiss Alps.

Letters from my father - March 1992:

> *Dear Cate,*
>
> *You may wonder why I have not made any comment to you on your illness. It is because I have been asked (by Jack) to keep out, and refrain from doing so. I have only really been able to say that I love you, which I say from the bottom of my heart.*
>
> *However, I am going to say this before I sign off. You have always been a positive person Cate, and on your own have made many decisions and achieved a great deal. You have helped many people to achieve, and helped their self-esteem. You have given yourself tirelessly and have really good values. Let us see the fruits once more.*

Be positive and remember that no matter what, we love you and that there is a huge amount of people who pray for you each day.

Lots of love, Dad

March 1992

My Darling Daughter,

... I must say quite clearly that you have been a real inspiration to me and a lot of other people in your lifetime. I have been thinking about some of those times like when you had the guts to stand up to your schoolteacher for your own beliefs in your own way. And when you ran the shop for Audrey at thirteen years old by yourself, at your own asking. How you decided to go to Tonga and how you saved your own money for it and went at your own volition.

How cross I was when they would not accept you for physiotherapy, and how glad I was when you qualified as a nurse - again, all by yourself and for yourself. Remember when you decided to go to Hamilton in your car just after you got your license? Pretty brave, huh? Another of your own decisions. Remember how keen you were to learn a brass instrument and how quick you learned? Another of your decisions. You really did make your own life you know.

I continually meet people who knew you as their nurse, or from when you worked at Bernina, or those people whom you helped. Like when you mentored Tania, who still carries your letter in her Bible. Your friends at the Gisborne corps all remember you, are praying for you, and send their love. You really only need to think back *to see that you lived your life as <u>you</u> wanted to, and people loved you for it.*

You have told me that you lived for others' expectations. I have searched my memories for that and find this not true. You have done lots of things for yourself and others out of love and compassion. This is why you have so <u>many</u> well-wishers. We all love you and I am the proudest. Just believe us. I could not tell you a lie, especially with so much at stake.

Well, I must close now. I am thinking of you. I do not expect anything of you except that you get better. We all love you and need you. Get well soon.

Love, Dad

Tuesday 17 March 1992
Jack and I saw my psychotherapist Carmia for the first time today. She intensely questioned Jack, and he was forced to defend himself. Carmia was not buying his excuses. It's the first time anyone has suggested that someone other than my parents could be the cause of my anorexia. Carmia is a stout and imposing Israeli-German woman. She was so forthright in examining Jack's role in my illness. No one had done this till now, and Jack was uncomfortably on the defensive.

Later, her words became a turning point in my understanding of my anorexia. But at the time, I strongly defended Jack! Carmia had then quit questioning Jack. Instead, my parents were summoned.

On several occasions, my parents traveled to Wellington for psychotherapy sessions with me and Carmia. These were difficult and painful experiences for them, and for me.

Nonetheless, Carmia was the best therapist I ever had. We remained friends until her death in 2023. She came to deeply regret she did not follow her instincts in pursuing Jack's part in my illness. At a certain point Jack's true colors became unmistakable.

Wednesday 18 March 1992

Jack and I went to Rebekah and Richard's home last night for dinner. I coped surprisingly well. It was the first meal I have eaten with people for a long time. Thankfully I was able to serve myself.

Rebekah and I spent some time together in the evening. Being such a good friend, I opened up to her about my dishonesty and stealing that had caused me so much guilt. She listened carefully, giving no verbal or non-verbal messages of shock or judgement. When she did speak, her words were gracious and loving. Wow, someone knows the worst of me and still seems to love me! The professionals who have been saddled with me don't count - they are paid to show care and tolerance.

I told Rebekah I needed comfort and encouragement. She told me that the original meaning of the word comfort was 'to give strength,' and to encourage was 'to give courage.' The words 'strength' and 'courage' seem far more powerful and suit me better.

Saturday 21 March 1992

A 'low' day from the beginning. It's not that things have gone wrong since being home, it's the difficulty of coping with things going right! Eating three meals a day, realistic exercise, prescribed laxatives only, and no 'reversing.' My mind continually opposes this behavior.

It is hard to escape the anorexic state of mind. I call it the 'Cruel Master.' It is the voice I have been listening to and believing. That voice still speaks to me, but now I have others; they say eat regular meals, moderate exercise, no bingeing and purging. I'm still getting use to all the contending voices. It's exhausting. It's like swimming against the tide. I am so tired of it. Sometimes all I can do is cry.

*****

There are very few things in life where you
do the right thing and it feels wrong,
but that's how it is with the recovery process
from an eating disorder.
As you go through the recovery process,
it just doesn't feel right,
and that's likely because the eating disorder
was serving some purposes for the patient,
particularly emotion regulation.
Michael Rollin, MD, Psychiatrist
- Eating Disorder Center of Denver

While the recovery stage is a positive step for someone with an eating disorder, it can't be assumed that quality of life will improve immediately. Some people with eating disorders struggle with the disease their entire life. Experts agree that recovery is an extremely challenging process not only for the patient but for supporting health professionals as well. Part of that is because individuals with an eating disorder often feel worse during the recovery than they did while struggling with the eating disorder. People with an eating disorder have a higher suicide risk during recovery.

*****

Sunday 22 March 1992
Tired and washed-out today from the emotional drain of yesterday. My eyes are still puffy and sore from crying. I went to Church this morning thinking it might help me. It didn't. It was unhelpful and inappropriate. Church seemed superficial and incapable of dealing with real problems. I feel isolated from all the people there. I am alone.

Monday 23 March 1992
Despite the difficulties and desperation of the past couple of days, my eating has held together. Technically it is a success, but I sure don't feel like it.

Tuesday 24 March 1992
I feel like I've taken my hands off the steering wheel of a car and the worst is going to happen. That is, to get fatter and fatter.

Jack brought me flowers today as an encouragement for "doing so well."

2024 Looking Back:
This was the devilish part of the disease I was engulfed in. Although my relationship with Jack had brought me to the point of suicide - I thought that I was no good and hopeless. He would then ride to the rescue and show his 'caring,' flowers, and cards, etc. I would even relay them to my therapists, family and friends. This elevated him in the eyes of everyone else.

I came to realize that much of it was for others to see, not for me. Jack wrote "I love you" on all the cards displayed on the mantle - yet I have no memory of him telling me. I have turned this over and over in my mind many times, and I cannot remember him ever saying to me, *"I love you."* He would write it, but not say it to me.

*****

Sunday 29 March 1992
There seems to be a conspiracy going on between the people I know, to tell me I am not fat even though I am. I am an emotional, mental and physical wreck as I struggle on my tight-rope. There seems no benefit from progress. Progress has slowed down.

I wish the people I ring for support just knew how things are for me at the time and how they can best support me. Invariably I end up having long and wearying conversations, only to gain a lesser measure of energy, encouragement and strength. This makes me reluctant to reach out despite how much I may need them. I feel like whatever or whoever is holding me up, is about to drop me.

Wednesday 1 April 1992
Why do I fear and hate looking like a woman? All I want is to look straight and non-gender slender. My increasing bust distresses me. I feel out of control. The eternal battle rages. The male body, particularly that of Jack, is off-putting to me. I no longer want sexual intimacy.

*****

2024 Looking Back:
I eventually began asking myself some rather obvious questions. Is Jack what I was reacting against? Was my weight loss and unattractive clothes a way of protecting myself from Jack's attentions? Why had I started wearing shapeless black clothing and boots all the time?

Jack shocked me one day when he led me into an Adult-Only Sex Shop. The windowless store was filled with all kinds of items I had never seen in my life before. That is because I had never been in such a store! I would have thought the same of Jack, my Salvation Army officer husband, except that he was showing and explaining numerous items to me that clearly, he knew about. I was naive, but not so naive that I could not recognize bondage and discipline paraphernalia, and seemingly every other conceivable option for indulging sexual fetishes. This was sexual degradation to me, and not a place I wanted to be.

It took my breath away and I wanted to leave, but Jack pressured me to stay and take it all in. I did so silently. This sex shop was on the same inner city street Jack worked on at The Salvation Army Headquarters. Did he have no shame that someone may have seen us go in there? I did! I remember thinking…. I bet Jesus did not walk in here with us! I told Jack I was not going back there again.

There was another time, while I was a patient at Ashburn Hall in Dunedin, Jack had traveled down to visit with me for a few days. He was given permission to take me on an outing, and it was to an Adult Only Store he took me. I had the same revulsion as the previous time.

I told him I did not want to go in, but I did not want to upset Jack or argue that I was denying him. Jack made a purchase of some clothing items and sex toys which he took home with him. I was again coerced into something sexually perverse.

*****

Thursday 2 April 1992

I went to Palmerston North today to see Dr. Andy. It was really good to see him. I told him how I should feel better with my progress, but I do not. The struggle is wearying. Life is kinder to me with no Exercycle and more freedom with food, but this creates other problems of guilt about my increasing weight.

I asked him when this blind-folded walk would end. When would I know for myself that what I do is right without having to blindly trust others. He could not tell me when, but believed it would begin to happen without my realizing it at first. As I was leaving, Dr. Andy told me that his first observation of me in the waiting area was that I was not wearing black for a change. He asked if this was a conscious or sub-conscious thing. I told him that I think it was conscious - that I felt different, so I wanted to look different. He then said he was never convinced that black suited me anyway!

Sunday 5 April 1992

I shocked myself and Patricia as we walked along the beach today. I began a sentence with *"when I get well..."* The possibility and desire of being well has been foreign to my mind. I'd had no thoughts about my future for some time now.

Wednesday 15 April 1992

Carmia asked me today why the self-destructive behavior became apparent while in The Salvation Army Training College? I told her I didn't really know.

2024 Looking Back:
This question might have cracked it all open if I'd had some insight. I still did not know there was anything wrong in my marriage, only that there was something wrong with me. Perhaps if Carmia had dug deeper. Jack's desire for control and the training regimentation seemed to fit like a hand in a glove. I got sicker and sicker with frightening speed. I began to fear not being able to conceive a child.

Instead, Carmia and I talked about how I make life hard for myself. I am back to my obsessive and compulsive swimming style - counting the number of lengths I swim, competing against the clock and other swimmers, and gaining satisfaction from seeing others rest or quit while I continue. My swimming will only have been worthwhile if I accomplish my quota and exhaust myself. Carmia felt that regardless of my objections I should instead go and do something kind for myself. But what does being kind to myself mean? How do I do it?

Thursday 16 April 1992
We had dinner at Rebekah and Richard's. Even eating with them is still far from straight-forward. In silent horror I watched Rebekah prepare the meal. The peas had salt! sugar! <u>and</u> butter! The carrots and broccoli were cooked in the wok with oil! and sauces! <u>Horror</u>! There were canned beets, along with a meat and vegetable pie that had flaky pastry! The lettuce and tomatoes were the only things I felt okay to eat. I did have a small piece of pie, which was delicious.

Food like this must be normal - as no apology was made for it - yet for me it makes eating no easy task. So much confusion and conflict. This is supposed to be a positive thing as it shows that there must be more than one possibility, more than one option.

It seems that life till recently has been like being on a rigidly straight, narrow, up-hill and non-negotiable highway. I came to a point of seeming destruction on this highway. In actual fact, it was a junction, and I have now chosen a different direction. My new direction has me on a road that offers me a lot more freedom.

In contrast to the old journey where I marched along an austere highway, it seems that this road could make my journey far more pleasant. I’m told that these strange and colorful things I see which possess 'fragrances,' are called flowers. What an unusual concept! I feel some guilt for stopping to smell the flowers, rest or look at wonderful things around me. Carmia tells me this is okay to do, and what the new road is about.

Carmia also tells me she’s seen me dancing instead of marching. I hadn't even realized! She said this is okay too. I do not yet feel far enough down this road to feel secure or safe. It’s still strangely unfamiliar.

The **‘shaft of light’** had brought about a big turnaround in me, but there was to be an even bigger incentive to recover.

This kind of woman, when paired with an emotionally
and spiritually healthy man, can co-create
a beautiful and powerful marriage.
But when a woman like this is paired with a toxic man
who believes he is entitled to power over women,
especially his own woman, a distorted
and sick version of marriage is birthed.
Natalie Hoffman - Is It Me

*****

When I reached the turning point, deciding I wanted to live and become well again, I began working to restore a normal body weight and establish normal eating habits. I was also anticipating that at some stage my monthly menstrual cycle would return. Prior to having anorexia, my menstrual cycle of every twenty-eight days was as regular as clockwork. With the starvation brought on by anorexia, that stopped. My womb was no longer a healthy and nutrient rich environment for a child to grow.

It was a huge surprise all round when just a short time after being discharged from the Wellington Psychiatric inpatient care, I immediately had two normal menstrual cycles, exactly twenty-eight days apart!

When the expected third menstrual cycle did not come on the twenty-eighth day, I was so disappointed. Food issues had started to become chaotic once more, and the lethargy that made me angry with myself resulted in throwing up food again. I was commenced on another course of anti-depressants in the hope of easing these symptoms. I felt angry with God that my period should be late when I was trying so hard. It seemed to put the possibility of pregnancy further from my reality, then… What was going on?

Could I be pregnant?

*****

Tuesday 2 June 1992

I left home at 12 noon with a urine sample to take to the doctors for a pregnancy test. The nearer I got to the Medical Centre the more nervous and sicker I felt. The practice nurse made small talk with me while waiting for the result. She also asked very tentatively if I wanted a 'positive' or 'negative.' "*It looks like a ... well, let's just wait till it is properly finished,*" she said. Then smiling, she passed the plastic square to me. Sure enough a positive was emerging. I could hardly believe it!

"Congratulations!" the nurse said in a very pleased but far too ordinary way. If she had known how desperately I had wanted to conceive and how miraculous and wonderful this pregnancy was, I am sure her response would have been far more overt. But this did not matter to me. I was ecstatic!

Having attempted to suppress any hope of pregnancy, I wasn't prepared for such news. I responded in a very controlled way by saying, *"Thank you. You have made my day."* No doubt if the reality had hit me then, I would have hugged and kissed her, and told her she had *"made my life!"* Finally, I have the permission to plan, dream and imagine.

I was twenty-eight years old, ecstatic and deeply grateful. I saw it as Yehovah's belief and trust in me. Though I still had my battles to face, I had an incredible motivation to eat well and exercise in moderation.

I walked to the swimming pool feeling both numb and elated. I kept taking the plastic square out of my pocket to check it still showed positive! I had to make sure I had not been tricked - that I had not dreamed it. I only swam for half an hour instead of my usual hour and a quarter. I did not want to over-do it!

Wednesday 3 June 1992

I decided to wait till after dinner last night to tell Jack the incredible news. I put too much celery in the dinner for Jack's liking and so he picked his way through it. I thought he would never finish! With only a small portion left on his plate, I could wait no longer. I handed him a note that said, *"congratulations, DAD!"* Of course he did not believe me. I had to prove it to him with the positive on my little plastic square. Jack was dumbfounded! Then, he was very happy.

We had to tell someone. We drove to Upper Hutt to share the news with Rebekah and Richard. I was not prepared for Rebekah's exacerbated assaulting embrace of joy that nearly broke ten of my ribs instead of the usual five! I said to Rebekah and Jack that I now had an excuse for being fat. Eyebrows were raised and Jack responded, *"Rome wasn't built in a day!"*

We were both so excited and happy. Neither of us could remember the last time we shared such a pleasant time together without argument or upset. I kept wondering if this was only a dream and I would soon wake up.

Pregnancy well explains the symptoms of recent weeks. I had been feeling super anxious about my increased weight and appetite, but now... well I still don't feel good about it, but there is a reason!

Jack tells me that while we were watching a television advertisement for Kentucky Fried Chicken the other night, he had a funny feeling, but quickly dismissed it, that I could be pregnant. I had said that I would really like to eat some. This could have been a normal response for almost anyone else, but extremely out of character for me. Was it a pregnancy craving? - he had wondered.

Thursday 4 June 1992

Today I have painted a terracotta pot to put my 'Cate' plant in. I am going to give it to Dr. Andy. I have also made a small flag to stick in the soil with the words, "Transformed by Grace."

When I run now, I am starting to feel something I don't want to feel. I will have to start wearing a bra again!

Saturday 6 June 1992

I am fearing my bed and sleep again. Being awake for long periods of time is lonely, tiring and stressful. Being in darkness is still frightening. I sometimes awaken needing to tell someone about the feelings that are disturbing me. I cannot speak to Jack about them. The reactions and attitudes I receive from others, often interfere with my journey. I do not connect emotionally with Jack. I cannot speak my mind.

Monday 8 June 1992

I was so stirred up at church yesterday. Why can't Christians be real about their problems so they can be real about the answers?

Today I had an appointment with Dr. Andy. I told him one of the things that concerned and panicked me about pregnancy was my clothing. In particular dresses. For me, pregnancy + summer = dresses.

I was distressed when trying maternity dresses on the other day. I looked prissy, nice, compliant, feminine and conventional, all things I was no longer interested in being. I told Dr. Andy how I had easily slipped into my image of jeans, baggy jerseys and boots, and that to slip out of it was hard. Dresses were a thing of my old world. Dresses were just not me anymore.

Patricia had commented to me at different times that she had never seen me wearing a dress. Will I feel as dramatically changed and uncomfortable to others as I will feel myself when I wear a dress? What will people say and think? The worst place to wear a dress would be at church!

Dr. Andy however did not think that dresses were an inevitable consequence of pregnancy. That I could continue wearing trousers. He encouraged me to talk about these feelings over the months ahead. I think he understood.

Another thing I talked with Dr. Andy about was going back to church for the first time last Sunday. I had found it inappropriate, unhelpful and oppressive. He felt I was wrong to take the view that I was the problem, since many people go to church and have similar feelings. I gave him my 'Cate plant,' the African Violet that had nearly died and returned to life, just like me. It was a momentous occasion for me and Dr. Andy!

Wednesday 10 June 1992
The whole issue of sex came up with Jack after dinner last night when he suggested we make love. I would have obliged despite not wanting to, but the conversation became too much for me. I felt pushed too far. As I lay face down in my usual escape place on the bedroom floor, I was almost totally unable to respond to Jack's attempts of communication. All I could do was nod, but even this was impossible when he asked me two questions at once! *"Can you not speak, or don't you want to speak?"*

Much later, I was finally able to talk. I told Jack that even what he had considered to be the most reasonable and minimal of requests, was too much for me.

The more he tries to make me realize how my lack of interest in sex affects him and how hard I am making it for him, the more guilty and inadequate I feel, and the more unable I am to function. The whole sex thing has become extremely difficult for me. It's hard enough to accept my own femininity and sexuality, let alone what being intimate with Jack means! Jack's continued expectations make me not want to have sex with him. Actually, I just don't want sex!

2024 Looking Back:
Jack's emotional abuse, by power and control over me, had led to this nightmare of self-degradation leading to anorexia. The obligation of marital intimacy brought out those very same feelings in me - inadequacy, fear and shame.

I did not want to be sexually attractive, dresses made me look more feminine, baggy trousers did not. We came to the agreement that Jack would only make his desire and need for sex known to me, and I will oblige as I feel able. He will be prepared to accept a *"no"* response from me. That intention was not borne out. Eventually, his desire for me to perform, not normal sex but *unwanted* sex acts with him, became coerced and insistent.

Friday 12 June 1992
Morning sickness again today. Jack keeps reminding me that I once said, *"I don't care how bad I feel when I am pregnant. I just want to be pregnant."* At least I am only feeling sick. I think I have done enough throwing up to last me a lifetime!

Saturday 13 June 1992
Another strange thing - I had a craving for something tangy like spaghetti for lunch. The thought of my ritualistic and safe rye bread sandwich with salad for filling was unappealing. We bought hot chips for supper while we were out tonight. I really enjoyed them. Jack was still hungry when we arrived home, yet to his amazement I told him that I felt satisfied. This must be the first time I have used this word. Guilt or anger thoughts usually prevail - certainly after bad foods - but today I was satisfied!

Sunday 14 June 1992
I still have troubling feelings about eating all these 'bad' foods, but generally I am enjoying this newfound freedom and permission. I am excited about eating nice things when we go to Australia. Another realization for me is that the two recent times I have had chips, I have been able to wait till we got to a nice place to eat them. Usually, I have to eat them immediately - so as to get the guilty pleasure over

and done with. Becoming pregnant gave me the opportunity and permission to eat a whole range of foods I had not allowed myself for a long time, certainly not without purging.

*****

Monday 15 June 1992
Mid-morning I made myself pancakes with prunes for breakfast. This response to food is freaky. Until now, I have not transgressed my morning ritual of bran and prunes. What is happening to me? Last night I ate sausages, mashed potato, beets, peas and corn! I'm amazed at my food choices. I even walked to town today and stopped along the way for a rest! Normally I would never let myself rest.

Thursday 18 June 1992
I talked to Jack's mother on the telephone tonight. She was delighted when I told her I had just eaten chocolate cake for supper. It was fortunate that she was sitting down when I then told her I had eaten a cream doughnut for lunch. I think she was quite shocked!

Sunday 21 June 1992
I have had another telephone conversation with Rebekah. I told her how my changing body shape is concerning to me. Anorexia had changed my body image. All I wanted to look like was straight up and down - like a boy. There is even less hope of this happening in the next nine months! My weight and size will be totally out of my control. She told me that over the past eighteen months I have looked like a young Italian boy. Rebekah thought that despite my boyish appearance, I had grace and elegance. Hmm. To me, being boyish was part of the goal to <u>not</u> be sexually attractive to Jack.

The pendulum swing of eating is bizarre! I need to experience the freedom of eating before getting to equilibrium. It is like not having to attend church services. It would not be enough just to be told that I did not have to go. I actually have to exercise my freedom and not go. In the same way, just to be told I have the freedom to eat the once forbidden foods is no freedom at all. I have to exercise this freedom. I owed it first and foremost to free myself to get better and live.

Thursday 25 June 1992
We've arrived at Surfer's Paradise, a wonderful beach north of Brisbane.

I didn't cope well with lunch today and my response to Jack led to another heated episode with him. All I really needed from him was encouragement and support about my eating, but he immediately launched into his savage and last-ditch attempt to get me to eat right. I had eaten with the most freedom I had ever had during the last two weeks. To Jack, the difficulties with food I was having again, was unacceptable.

Saturday 27 June 1992
It was a bad start to the day when I decided to wear my white trousers. I was freaked out at how tight they felt. This led to a great argument and upset with Jack that lasted three quarters of an hour. Instead of him accepting what I was saying and feeling, he attempted yet again to dictate my feelings. It makes me so mad when Jack rationalizes my feelings away.

Tuesday 21 July 1992
We're having a girl! The scan of the baby today showed that everything is well.

Thursday 23 July 1992
It was a useful session with Dr. Andy. I talked with him about Jack and sex. Since the functional task of becoming pregnant had been achieved, having sex had now become worse for me. I was unable to work out why my attitude and response to sex had changed so dramatically since being unwell. I feel like a bad wife! Dr. Andy opined that such an outcome was reasonable considering the emotional trauma of the past eighteen months.

He also thought it was reasonable to be given space by Jack. Jack and Dr. Andy had both arrived at the conclusion of 'time out,' but their rationales were different. Jack sounds righteous but I sense the message beneath it that he is offended, even outraged, that his marital right to sex is being taken away. This creates guilt for me, and I'm left believing I’m being unreasonable and rejecting Jack. Dr. Andy, however, acknowledges the trauma of recent times and the need I have for 'time out' regardless of the inconvenience to Jack. He allows me to believe I have a right to my feelings and needs, and that resolution will only come when no expectations are on me.

Tuesday 4 August 1992

Susan is back in hospital. She’s suicidal again. I am on the edge of feeling guilty and apologetic that I am now getting better, am pregnant, and my life may appear 'sweet' to her. Valorie suggests that I consider myself as a picture of hope for Susan. Yes. When I was that depressed, what I needed was a friend who could tolerate my pain and despair, and bring me hope. I feel so much compassion and love for Susan.

Sunday 9 August 1992

Progress is like the ebb and flow of the tide. I often wonder if it’s reasonable for me to need so much therapy help.

Monday 10 August 1992

I wonder about God. I am told that He’s unchanging, all-powerful and loving, but why is it that He seems passive in His involvement at one time and dynamically active at another? Why is it that often only in retrospect can we recognize His presence in a crisis situation?

Is it only me that can’t experience His consistent presence? Has God been playing games with me? Why is it that I do not seem capable of understanding His role in my life?

Thursday 13 August 1992

My daily walks are becoming more enjoyable. I think the improving weather is a big factor, but mainly because I’m not driving myself to burn calories. There are now times when I will stop to smell an early spring flower or pause along the Ridgeway to appreciate the view. I often stop at the Ridgeway Park and will swing on a swing. I do a lot of thinking here. I also talk to my baby, Ruby.

Friday 14 August 1992
I visited Susan at the hospital again today. The weather was cool and grey but we sat out in the courtyard so she could smoke, and we could have some privacy. Although her concentration level was poor, we did talk about perfectionism and my experience of becoming well.

*****

Until 24 February 1992, life for me was like fighting a fierce gale! That had led to my second attempt at suicide. I acquired the plant that I call my 'God plant' when God saved me from death. It was only when I reached my turning point in Ward 27 at Wellington Hospital, that I became aware the growth of these three flowers on my 'God plant' represent God's grace and mercy, and redemption.

For You have delivered my soul from death.
Have You not kept my feet from falling,
That I may walk before God
In the light of the living?
Psalm 56:13

As I started to realize how God had miraculously intervened to save my life, I determined that from then on, my testimony to others of what God was like would be nothing more and nothing less than this encounter with Him. I had experienced something of this grace, mercy and redemption when He proved His willingness and desire to have me live. I certainly could not understand why He would want to save a hopeless scumbag like me, but the fact was He did. I decided that if this was all I ever knew about God, this was okay. I was not going to generate or create anything. I was still unable to grasp anything of God's love.

Often, I would watch people slouch over in their seats— perhaps because of guilt and condemnation. People would walk into the church building laughing and smiling and leave appearing quite despondent. Mixed messages were frequently given. For example, everyone would sing a song about how God's love could not be earned by our own good efforts, and the next minute someone from the platform would be pressuring people into being committed and fulfilling their Godly duties!

I much preferred to be with non-Christians who were attempting to be real in their sufferings. Among them I felt much more honest and able to be my authentic self. The church seldom helped me on my quest for reality. In my more rational and objective times, I surmised that the church must be a poor representation of Yehovah.

2024 Looking Back:
My experience of church was confusing and separating and I came to feel like a spiritual fugitive. I am sure I was overly critical at times; judging others in ways I did not want to be judged myself. For this I have repented. I did later learn that one in four marriages in the church have experienced physical, sexual or emotional abuse. So, many in the church do wear masks over their real selves.

Sunday 10 January 1993
Susan visited me this afternoon. I have come to love and care for her deeply. Susan's weight was the lowest it has ever been. She was extremely emaciated. Her appearance was heart wrenching. Susan serenely told me that she was going to die. She no longer wanted to live. She had no will to go on. It was too hard to cope with another day. Her manner was so like mine when I had walked the golf course with Rebekah prior to my second suicide attempt.

I had known this pain and despondency all too well. I could now better appreciate what others may have felt for me, and the difficult position I put Rebekah in when I required her silence.

In the two hours I had with Susan, I assured her of my continued love. I also told her that I did not want her to die, and that my conviction and experience was that while there is breath, there is hope.

2024 Looking Back:
Susan displayed what Satan had done. The same thing I had allowed

Satan to do to me - ***to steal, kill and destroy***, as stated in John 10:10. Satan attacks us to take away our ability to choose, and by so doing disqualify us. However, Yeshua came ***to give life, and that we may have it more abundantly***, as also stated in John 10:10.

Although Susan had not vowed me to secrecy, I knew that Susan had assumed this of me. I broke her confidence. I was not going to let my friend die.

Susan got through this crisis time and bought a small broken-down house. She totally renovated it, and in the process, got well. Several years after this particular visit with Susan I attended her wedding. She was a beautiful bride! With the help of a good man, she completely overcame anorexia. She also had two children and returned to work as a Registered Nurse.

TREASURE BEYOND COMPARE

Every good gift and every perfect gift is from above,
coming down from the Father of lights,
with whom there is no variation or shifting shadow.
James 1:17

The promise to Abraham was the blessing to him that his seed would proliferate like the stars in the sky. The greatest blessing of Yehovah - is to bless His people with descendants!

Tuesday 9 February 1993
At 11:44 pm yesterday Ruby was born, weighing 3.380 kilograms - 7 lbs 5 oz.

I do not know what I was expecting to come out, but I was certainly surprised when I saw it was a baby! My fears about her well-being were unrealized, as she is just perfect. Ruby is my miracle!

The pain of childbirth is far exceeded by the joy I feel, as I have been holding Ruby in my arms! I am wondering if the suddenness and speed at which she came, is going to be indicative of an impetuous, impatient and determined personality. And indeed, it was!

Ruby's dedication on Sunday 8 March 1993 was a very significant event. In dedicating her to Yehovah, Jack and I also wanted to acknowledge our daughter as being a beautiful gift of Yehovah's grace to us.

This occasion was made even more special by the many friends and family members who joined with us. Yes, happily for me, Mum and Dad were there. Over fifty people had merged with the usual church group, making the church hall very full of excited noise and bodies. Among these fifty, were those who shared the anorexia road with me. Susan was one of them. There were also those who had been, and continued to be, key people in my journey to life and wholeness. It seemed not only right that they should be there, but also that some of them take part.

Carmia read an appropriate Scripture passage in Hebrew, Rebekah prayed for Ruby, Ed sang her a beautiful song of blessing, and Dr. Andy gave a Bible message about our perceptions of Yehovah and the realities of living. This of course had significance to the road I had travelled. It was Patricia who performed the actual dedication of Ruby.

Among the things Patricia spoke, was her remembrance of the 24th of February 1991 which was the day she and Ed first met Jack and I. Life was bleak and confusing. The 24th of February 1992 was the day she had visited me in Wellington Hospital's Intensive Care Unit. Then on the 24th of February 1993 she had visited Jack, Ruby and I in our home.

*****

Monday 17 May 1993

Dear Ruby,

It is Monday 3:30 pm and you are sitting on my knee at the dining room table. I thought I would write you a letter on this piece of paper I have just painted. A letter to tell you again how much I love you.

You continue to bring us much joy and laughter (and wakeful nights!). You are growing up so fast. No longer are you the tiny helpless newborn babe I held in my arms three months ago. Every day your personality and individuality become more evident. A beautiful and precious person is developing before my eyes - like a tiny bud coming into flower. How well will my memory serve me in years to come?

Will I remember your lovely little face with its many interesting expressions, your delightful noises, your soft tiny hands that love to hold, touch, and be sucked, the sound of your cries that alert me to your needs, your perfectly formed little body - ever increasing in mobility, strength and skill, and of course your most charming and endearing smile. Especially that first one!

As this bud unfolds
May I always
Protect and appreciate its beauty
I love you Ruby

Despite the struggles I continued to have after the birth, Ruby proved to be very much a part of my healing process. I did not seem to crash as frequently. When I did, I often got over it quicker. Sometimes it was Ruby's smile or just her very presence that would lift me. In a sense, she became 'Emmanuel' - which means 'God with us' - to me.

It was like Yehovah expressed His approval and encouragement to me through her.

Of course, with the delights of having a new-born came the weariness. Ruby was not a baby that would lie quietly or sit and watch the world go on around her. She was hard work. She wanted to be in on all the action, which meant carrying or holding her constantly. The purchase of a Jolly Jumper at five months saved me. She stood unaided at fifteen weeks, crawled at six months and was walking at nine months.

Ruby was also sleep-resistant. Jack and I consequently discovered numerous ways of rocking and juggling her hammock to get her to sleep at night. Success was when we could get her to sleep after only two hours of vigorous motion! It was not infrequent for Ruby and I to be up playing together from three or four in the morning. Although Ruby started eating solids at seven months, she much preferred her ever-frequent breast feeding. We shared many special times together in the day and night hours as I nursed her.

I was always so proud to take her out. With the pram or the back-pack, we walked many a mile together. I especially liked our Saturday or Sunday afternoon walks along Oriental Parade, where we joined countless other pram-pushing-parents.

Thursday 2 December 1993

> *Dear Ruby.*
>
> *You will be ten months old in one week's time. You have won our hearts in a BIG way. I cannot imagine what life would now be like without your presence, and the love and joy you bring.*
>
> *Words seem inadequate to describe the depth of love I have for you. There are many times I sit and look at you. When you are busily playing, snuggled into me asleep, when we are enjoying a swim or a bath*

together, or when you are happily babbling away on the change table. My heart pulsates with indescribable love for you.

Our family dynamics have not been so pleasant again lately. The need I feel to lose weight has become very important again. You seem to sense and react to the tension this creates. Is your perception as acute as I fear?

It is difficult enough for me to understand and cope, so I imagine it must be harder for you.

I feel quite torn between the obsession to control my weight, and my love for Daddy and you. One side will ultimately win.

God, please let it be Jack and Ruby.

2024 Looking Back:
I realize it was this fear of losing my husband and now my child, my family, that held my anorexia in place. Jack's oft-repeated statement was that if I ever got well, I would leave him behind.

*****

CHAPTER 5

Pharaoh - The Cruel Master

Pharaoh charged all his people, saying,
Every Hebrew son that is born -
You shall cast into the river!
Exodus 1:22

Sunday 16 August 1992
The first Salvation Army event I attended after a long absence was last night. It proved to be a similar experience to the following scenario:

> *...you've changed the scenery; you've moved onto the second act, so to speak, and you're afraid that by going back to the old setting from the first act, you might fall into your old role. Being surrounded by the same old scenery and acting with the same old characters might cause you to read the same old lines since that's all you've known to do in that environment.*
> **Cherry Boone O'Neill** - Starving for Attention

Monday 17 August 1992
When I visited Susan in hospital today, I was reminded of an art day at school in standard one (elementary). We crayoned layer upon layer of different colors on a piece of card, finishing with a top layer of black. We then scratched out a picture and saw the under colors emerge. This seemed to symbolize my friend's present state of blackness, yet with glimpses of color starting to emerge.

Although I resent Jack attempting to get things under control for me, I am also aghast how dependent I am on Jack to protect me from myself. My attempts to declare my freedom, although often inappropriate and self-destructive, result from the ongoing inner conflicts; with food, with myself, and with Jack.

Friday 30 October 1992
I always perceive my increased weight and fat as the problem. They are the scapegoat for every hurt, misunderstanding, and conflict. I am realizing that this eating disorder is my solution to the whatever the problem is, however inappropriate.

Thursday 6 May 1993
I have had a couple of bad days. The bottom-line has been self-hatred, and all the baggage that goes with it - depression, condemnation, guilt, fear, wanting to hurt myself, and a diminished sense of freedom.

My mind-set has become anorexic again!

2024 Looking Back:
I had not overcome or even figured out the controlling influence of Jack, or the controlling influence of Satan's lies - both of which were defining my belief about who I was. Pregnancy had interrupted this issue. Now it was once again an issue.

I was letting Jack and Satan define who I was. I was not looking to Yeshua to define who I was.

If I were to counsel someone in a similar predicament now, I would show them in the Bible what our loving Creator says about them and how He feels towards them. I would encourage them to write out verses like: 2 Corinthians 5:17, Romans 8:38-39, Psalm 139:13-14, Ephesians 2:10, and 1John 3:1, and to read these out loud regularly throughout the day, until truth overcomes the lies.

I would also encourage thankfulness, because being thankful increases dopamine - a natural chemical in the brain - which allows us to see and understand the Truth.

*****

Self-hatred had an insatiable appetite. It was not enough just for me to hate myself. I wanted others to hate me too. Self-hatred was a downward spiral. It created the desire to eat and purge. More self-hatred followed, bringing feelings of anger, disgust and failure, and so fueling the fire for another round.

2024 Spiritual Awakening:
In my time of anorexia, as I starved, binged and purged and exercised punishingly – I lost sight of my true self and of my body being the temple of the Holy Spirit. So instead of glorifying Yehovah with my body I was desecrating Yehovah's Temple. To desecrate is to violate the sanctity of the Temple by treating it irreverently and contemptuously. I did so under the duress of the Cruel Master – Satan!

***Or do you not know that your body is the temple of the Holy Spirit who is in you**, whom you have from God, and you are not your own? For you were bought at a price; therefore glorify God in your body and in your spirit, which are God's.*
1 Corinthians 6:19-20

Over time, as I accepted myself as the Temple of Yehovah - I came to see that one does not desecrate the Temple - or let others do so through sexual and domestic abuse, drugs or Electroshock. I had to switch from Satan's lies to Yehovah's truth. Of course, Satan wanted me hyper-focused on my weight and my failures as a woman, wife, and mother. He did not want me seeing myself as the precious holder of the Holy Spirit. Although I was raised in the church, I had no idea how Satan worked through manipulating our emotions and failings, the open doors we leave for him to enter and attempt to control us. What was Yehovah's agenda for me and for my body?

Yeshua - when he found money changers defiling the Temple for profit - drove them out with force. Yehovah - when the Greeks defiled the Temple by sacrificing a pig - sparked a rebellion among the Israelites. This is in the Book of Maccabees. Imagine that - rather than allow a sacrilegious sacrifice to be made and eaten in his Holy Temple - Yehovah had the people rise up against the mightiest earthly empire in the world at that time, that of the Selucid Greeks. As a result, the Israelites became the strongest military force in the Middle East, fighting with the Angels of Yehovah going before them and recapturing all the territory of Israel since the time of David and Solomon. If my body is being used for ill - then Yehovah wants me to retake His territory.

How we treat our body and allow others to treat it - does matter enormously - Yehovah takes this with the utmost seriousness. I had yet to learn this lesson.

*****

Monday 10 May 1993

Having lived through a two-week emotional roller-coaster ride, I saw Carmia again. I came away feeling somewhat liberated by gleaning some new insights. Jack and I most often will not connect when I start to spiral downward. His anger and frustration are directed towards me. I resent this response, yet at the same time I expect it, and rely on it as a confirmation of the guilt and self-hate that I feel. Jack does the thinking for me. I need to do my own thinking and reasoning.

Saturday 5 June 1993

It is easier, in a sense, to maintain a chronic eating disorder. Although it is bondage and oppression, at least the rules, rigidity and structure of the eating disorder are known, which gives a sense of security. I know what is expected and how to play the game. To try and get out of the rut is harder. What are the rules for that? What can I expect? Why does it still feel so bad when I am trying to do the right thing? The goal of wellness seems elusive.

Most often I am thriving on the challenge of being a mother and keeping the house, but exercise is still my justification for eating.

20 June 1993

Susan visited this morning. In exchange for helping her make a card - she gave me a foot massage. This is the first one I have had, and it was a very emotional experience for me.

24 June 1993

Jack's natural response to most things is analytical. So when I feel like an awful, disgustingly obese person - Jack lectures me. His detached response reinforces how untouchable I feel. It reinforces the rejection. If I ask him to hold or touch me, it does not feel convincing - he will touch me - but not with his heart.

I do not know why my overwhelming self-hatred exists. When I believe myself to be disgusting and obese, I created that image in my mind. Apparently, it is not what others see.

It is not the image in the looking glass
that matters most,
but how that image reflects back
into the mind's eye.
Rita Freeman - Body Love

If a nail is hammered into a piece of wood a couple of times, it will come out relatively easily. However repeated hammering makes it extremely difficult to pull out. Since marrying Jack, I have pounded that nail with self-directed anger, accusations and assaults. Now, it has become a difficult nail to remove.

Because she is so committed to taking personal responsibility,
when he blames her for her supposed role
in his own bad behaviors,
she accepts the blame and works hard
to do better next time in order to avoid the guilty
and shameful emotions that follow an abusive incident.
This is perfect for him... Once he controls how
she defines his abuse of her, then he can control her actions.
Natalie Hoffman - Is It Me?

I need to put sandbags down to stop the destructive feelings flooding in and washing away the ground I have gained. I am told that poor body image has little to do with how I actually look, and that there is a strong relationship between body image and self-esteem i.e. the better my feeling of self worth - the better my body image. Apparently ,the mind dominates matter when it comes to body image, and body image and self-esteem are highly interdependent.

A basic premise of cognitive therapy is that your thoughts influence how you feel. Cognitive errors can have a big impact on body image. Some cognitive errors are: extreme thinking, rejecting positives, thinking in shoulds, personalizing, jumping to conclusions, emotional reasoning.
Rita Freeman - Body Love

2024 Spiritual Awakening:

Casting down arguments and every high thing that exalts itself against the knowledge of God, ***bringing every thought into captivity to the obedience of Yeshua Messiah****.*
2 Corinthians 10:5

*****

Wednesday 15 September 1993
I am at a cross-roads. I have felt an inner strength in recent weeks that is helping me take control of my body again. Till now I have not been happy with my eating and weight. This cannot be freedom. I want to try the 'healthy' way again, but this time get it right. I'm not confident though that I can. The potential for disaster is frightening. Exercising more and eating only 'healthy' approved foods could go too far.

The good things I now have in my life have only been found away from anorexia, and if I choose the anorexia way again, I could lose all the good things in my life. Although I am on the path to freedom - I have not got there yet. That's certain!

My mind still goes into over-load when I see an array of indulgent food. I may be eating all types of food now, but I am breaking all my rules. It makes me feel like a criminal!

Sunday 19 December 1993

My actions and reactions are a downward spiral, and could lead us back to where we were at three years ago. What a guilt trip! I love my family and do not want to hurt or lose them. I am living on a knife edge. My weight has dropped significantly again. My food intake is not good, and exercise takes up a good portion of my day.

I saw Dr. Caitlin, my psychiatrist, at the hospital on Wednesday. She seemed quite concerned about me. She even said I was too underweight. Hardly - I have so much fat! I am not feeling the depression of times gone by, but moments come when life seems too much again. I do not feel depressed, but my world is depressed. Dr. Caitlin believes I have a masked depression, and she has prescribed a different course of anti-depressants for me.

Ruby keeps me from spiraling downward even more. If there was only me, and no one else mattered, losing weight would become an all-consuming task. But there really is so much to lose, so much at stake. My inner resources are depleted. I sometimes feel resentful and angry to be woken too early in the mornings when I just want to crash out and sleep.

2024 Spiritual Awakening:

Stand fast therefore in the liberty by which Yeshua the Messiah has set us free, and do not be entangled again with a yoke of bondage.
Galatians 5:1

In Numbers 14:1-4 The Israelites complained, *"Let us appoint a leader to take us back to Egypt!"* The people were on the border of the Promised Land and had not the strength or faith to enter. They were fearful, neither was this the first time they wanted to return to bondage. It was simply incomprehensible - having reached the Promised Land which was the place of their inheritance! Faith is critical to our freedom from bondage. Freedom is the great unknown. We do not know what challenges await us. Bondage we know. **Freedom is also our inheritance!**

Getting free of anorexia was a long process for me, a roller coaster of failures and successes. As with the Israelites, the fear of letting go of the familiar bondage was overwhelming.

*****

Saturday 25 December 1993
Susan's early visit, and then watching Ruby open her Christmas presents, are the only things I have enjoyed about the day. Once we left the house this morning my worst fears were realized. I hate Christmas as it is so food orientated. The food is fatty, disgusting and way over the top. My mind suffers a horrible beating each Christmas Day!

I am set upon by fear, guilt, condemnation, chaos, confusion, shame, and hopelessness. The merriment continues around me, and no one sees my torment.

Monday 3 January 1994
Old patterns are increasingly being reinstated to my life. I put more and more rules and regulations upon myself, my eating, my exercise. I have surprisingly maintained my weight over the Christmas period. I was sure I had eaten way too much.

I have seen Dr. Caitlin again. She and Carmia are my only meaningful contacts. Rebekah and Valorie are all busy and out of the picture. I am living a sparse existence. The focus of each day is food, weight, exercise and Ruby. I have no energy or motivation to write, create, visit or telephone anyone. Getting through each day is an achievement. My only enjoyment comes from time with Ruby. All I want to do is sleep. It is only Ruby who gives my life any meaning or purpose. Her life and existence exemplify grace and freedom. I love her deeply.

I don't feel anything spiritual. The times I go to church I am irritated and bored. I feel like a con artist as I am so far away and separated from God. If not for Ruby...

Tuesday 4 January 1994
I cannot trust myself with food. Experience proves that once I start, I want to eat more. I am terrified of being out of control. I need to get off this treadmill, but the consequences are too scary. Why do people persist in giving chocolates and sweets to me at Christmas? Are they being vindictive, or just plain ignorant? My feelings of not being understood are ignited! In addition, I have to cope with the torment of too much holiday temptation.

Wednesday 5 January 1994
Just as Ruby needs a play pen at times to give her boundaries, keep her safe, and give security, **Jack thinks I also need a pen.** He tells me that when it comes to taking care of, and looking after myself, I display little wisdom, sense or maturity. I listen to my mind rather than my body. Until I can listen to and understand my body, perhaps I do need imposed constraints. For example, what is sensible and reasonable exercise? Jack is happy to dictate those constraints. When I cannot live up to them, I feel so guilty and worthless, like I am betraying my family. I am failing them.

Thursday 13 January 1994
Fear stops me going forward, and fear stops me going back. However, the grip of anorexia is getting stronger. Dr. Caitlin suggests I try to see the anorexia as a presence, and to externalize it. The Cruel Master is an image that fits for me.

Friday 28 January 1994
I believe what the Cruel Master tells me. This Master of mine is condemning, controlling, disrespectful, oppressing and humiliating. I must externalize Him and see His power over me. It immediately

reminded me of Catherine Cookson's movie *The Black Velvet Gown.* The character Biddy was sold into slavery to a cruel Master.

I must learn to see this Cruel Master as separately as I saw the Master in the film - so I can be assertive with him and true to myself. I feel like a caged animal!

Monday 7 February 1994
I have had a swollen and painful ankle for a few weeks now. Today I went to the doctor as it has gotten to the point where I cannot bear the weight of it or even touch anything without acute pain. The diagnosis is a repetitive strain injury from over exercising. I have been put on anti-inflammatory drugs. I am told that I need to give my foot complete rest for at least a week, and then to gradually introduce exercise. I dissolved into tears when he told me this! Already the pain had meant minimal exercise! How can I eat if I cannot exercise?

Tuesday 15 February 1994
The Cruel Master's strategy is for him to be merged into my personality so that he cannot be seen or detected. His insidious influence and control over me is a reflection of my personality. He cannot be beaten until he is exposed. The Cruel Master keeps the momentum of the pendulum swing going from restrictive control to over-eating. I need to beat him at his own game. Whether I am in the restrictive or over-eating mode, I need to take charge and assert myself. I need to resist and defy the Cruel Master.

2024 Spiritual Awakening:

That they may come to their senses
and escape the snare of the Devil,
having been taken captive by him to do his will.
2 Timothy 2:26

The Cruel Master was real! And he had taken me captive. We cannot defeat an enemy that we have not exposed. However, it took me years to see that the Cruel Master was another guise of Satan. He is the father of lies, the master of subterfuge. My therapy was bound to fail.

I was being treated for “Mommy” problems. Even if they had focused on Jack’s ill influence – the problem was still deeper than that. It was Satan who had snuck into my psyche – due to my naïveté – and planted the seeds of my destruction. It was Satan who took Jack’s sick influence, the therapists’ misdirection, the medication’s mind-numbing effects and wove them into a catastrophic masterpiece.

It is the truth that sets us free, and my fear was keeping me from truth. Satan is vicious but he does not have to be victorious. "*Greater is Yeshua who is in me - than Satan who is in the world!*” 1 John 4:4

*****

Just as Ruby will turn and run to me when I tell her in a gruff playing voice "*I'm coming to get you,*” I need to turn and face the Cruel Master instead of letting him chase me all the time. The issue is not about whether I eat or not. It is about making the choice in freedom. I need to start learning to hear my own voice and decide for myself, rather than letting the Cruel Master dictate. I need to assert my control and choice about eating, exercise etc.

2024 Looking Back:
It is true that Satan *cannot be beaten until he is exposed*, but also emotional and sexual abuse cannot be beaten until it is recognized, and exposed. I had still not identified it as such and was forbidden by Jack to speak of our relationship. Most all of my references to Jack in therapy were to exonerate him from blame or portray him as my devoted husband, my savior. So I had misidentified both the real Cruel Master and my true Savior. Not until later, when I was advised to go to a Women’s Refuge and received sexual abuse counseling, did I comprehend that what had happened to me was abusive. At first, I felt like a fraud being there.

*****

Friday 18 February 1994
My weight has increased by 1.5 kilograms, more than three pounds! I am panicked, but surprised it is not more, since I have been unable to exercise, and my eating has been excessive.

Friday 25 February 1994
I was super anxious prior to the session I had with Carmia and my mother yesterday. Carmia asked me what I had gained from the session. The only thing I could think about was my mother saying I was the daughter she and my father had hoped for. Having had two boys, they were so happy to have a little girl. Although the two and a half hours were emotionally exhausting for me, I saw them as being constructive. Carmia helped us to look at the relationship Mum and I had now and for the future. Not just reliving past regrets and failures.

2024 Spiritual Awakening:
There is a perfectly good reason we cannot go back in time with the knowledge we have now to correct a thing… it is Yehovah who does The <u>Work</u>.

Monday 28 February 1994
Today was another lengthy session. This time seeing Carmia with Mum and Dad. As we waited in the waiting area, I felt my world to be even more threatened with the presence of them both there. The psychiatric unit and the out-patient area had been my world - private from them. Today Mum and Dad were like intruders, and my old feelings of being a 'nutter' emerged once more. Although I had asked them to come, I now resented their presence.

It was another insightful time for me, but again I needed time to assimilate the two and a half hours' worth of therapy. Dare I hope that the measure of awareness we've each gained can make any on-going difference to our relationships?

2024 Looking Back:
The constant therapeutic blame put upon my parents had caused me to resent and condemn Mum and Dad beyond reason.

Most eating disorders have a sense of addiction to them,
and their purpose is often self-medicating.
For example, underneath most eating disorders
is a pretty severe depression.
Lerner, MD

Monday 17 October 1994
Dr. Sally, another psychiatrist I see at Wellington Hospital, has telephoned me each week-day because of her concern for my safety. The option of another admission to the psychiatric unit was therefore the main topic of conversation between Jack, her and I this morning. It all happened so quickly. I was given the last bed in ward 27.

*****

The fact that his words and actions don't match
make the experience all the more confusing,
throwing the victim into the depths of self-doubt.
Her religious community tell her she can't trust her heart.
It is "deceitful above all things."
They tell her she is making assumptions,
and this plays into her abuser's narrative.
These beliefs are implanted deep within her psyche now,
making it hard for her to tell right from wrong
when it comes to her own experiences.
Natalie Hoffman - Is It Me?

WARD 27

Wednesday 19 October 1994
My head is in turmoil as I try to work out what is happening to me and if the decision to be in hospital is the right one. Did I agree to this? Or am I agreeing because Jack and Dr. Sally think it is the right thing to do? Am I failing Ruby? How much does she understand?

Does she know that I love her? Please God keep Ruby safe, well and happy. Do not let her suffer because of me!

Although I had been back to the ward a number of times since my last admission, walking back into the ward as a patient again created unanticipated feelings of shame and embarrassment. I was angry with myself for feeling these things. My other feelings were uncertainty, confusion and relief.

Thursday 20 October 1994

There are so many doctors and nurses to talk with. Of course I want to be known and understood so I can be better supported, but being asked the same old questions over and over is tedious and irritating.

Feelings do not always have words. My need is for a sparse and disheveled environment. Unlike other times, I do not want flowers, cards, color or beauty. My unmade bed and scattered belongings make my cubicle area uncharacteristically untidy. Tidiness, order and beauty have expectations and responsibilities attached. I do not want the responsibility of keeping the flowers looking nice. I do not want to see them deteriorate. I do not want to see them die.

Saturday 22 October 1994

On admission my 'weapons,' scissors, razor, tweezers and clippers, were taken from me. They over-looked my small mirror!

I have been testing how safe this environment is for me since being here. To know if this place is any safer for me than being at home. Nursing staff insist on checking my mouth to ensure the tablets they give me have been swallowed. I cannot feel safe, and I am not safe, with myself, when I know I can deceive people who are supposed to be keeping me safe. For the same reasons I have concealed my mirror and have eaten virtually nothing for the last two and a half days.

Sunday 23 October 1994

With a head ready to burst last night, I finally got to talk with my nurse. We decided that talking time is to be negotiated each duty shift. Having arrived at this arrangement, I told her that *"Life is too bloody hard!"* She agreed with me, so I asked her if she enjoyed life. She replied very curtly - *"Mind your own business!"* - and that this had nothing to do with our interaction. I told her that I was sure it did have much to do with our interaction. What hope could she offer me if she had none herself? Before walking out on her, I asked her if she was so separate and removed that she could not even give a simple answer. I have also upset at least one other nurse. This came after I had thrown my partly done jigsaw all over the floor.

I returned to the ward at about 4:00 pm today having been for a drive around the bay with Jack and Ruby. We parked at Oriental Parade and I saw people walking to and fro. How do they do it? How do they all manage to cope with, and even enjoy life? I felt like an intruder in their world - someone strangely different.

Once back on the ward, I sat on the floor in an isolated corner for at least an hour and a half just staring at the wall. The only company I had was the confusion, agitation, rejection and self-hatred that tightly embraced me. I was feeling desperate and unsafe.

Monday 24 October 1994

I am thirty years old and I have just been angry with my mother (on the telephone) for the first time ever. My parents had rung and spoken to Jack late last night and, according to Jack, been disrespectful to him. My parents felt they had the right to know I was in hospital as soon as I was admitted, and that my mother could be looking after Ruby at this time.

Jack had been spoken to as if he were the villain and the cause of all my problems. They believed they knew me better than Jack did, and they knew what would be best for me. I was angry that my parents had opposed Jack and his actions towards me. They acted like they know something that I don't know.

2024 Spiritual Awakening:

Honor your father and your mother,
that your days may be long in the [Promised] Land
which Yehovah your God is giving you.
Exodus 20:12

So, it seems there is a pre-requisite for prospering in the Promised Land. Honor your parents. On a deeper, spiritual level - we are given a household with our Holy Father, to live in his loving relationship where he protects and prospers us as his children whom he never forsakes. It is the primary goal of Satan to break this bond, first with our earthly parents who are our model for our relationship with our Heavenly Father - then breaking the bond with Yehovah himself - removing ourselves from his blessing and protection by our own hand. Satan cannot do this unless we let him of our own free will.

The Promised Land is more than simply a physical place to put down seeds and put up houses. It is a place where we can freely serve our Creator. *"Yehovah, God of the Hebrews (those who 'cross over') says, 'Let My people go that they may freely serve Me!"* (Exodus 7:16). That is where our prosperity and blessing come from - our covenant promise with Yehovah. *"Remember, Yehovah your God, for it is He who gives you ability to get wealth, that he may establish His covenant which he swore to your fathers."* (Deuteronomy 8:18)

My parents knew a whole lot that I didn't know! How did I get things so back to front? How did I not see Jack for who he was and my parents for who they were? At that point, I was unaware of what a trauma bond was, and that this had developed between Jack and I. [See Chapter 9: *Stars in the Heavens* - for a deeper understanding of trauma bonding.]

*****

Monday 31 October 1994

As I sit looking out the window, I see a spindly green tree being battered by the fierce wind, rain and cold. It is unsupported and alone. The unrelenting onslaught of the wind causes it to remain bent right over. How much more of this treatment can it take? I cry, because despite the tree's obvious vitality and suppleness, it will break if the raging elements persist. I cry because the significant growth and change in me is not enough to withstand the unrelenting emotional elements that rage within me. I too lack the protection and the support that I need. When will I break?

It's important to pay attention to whether an individual
has a condition that predates the eating disorder,
such as depression, as eating disorders
have a high occurrence of co-morbidities.
In these cases, the issues regarding the eating disorder
may be resolved, but the preexisting condition
will continue or possibly worsen,
particularly if the eating disorder helped a patient
cope with the original condition.
Dr. Lerner - Clinical Psychologist

Tuesday 1 November 1994

Last night I had all my coat hangers taken away from me. I was on suicide watch. An evening of intense self-hatred left me in no fit state to see any visitors. I think the nurse told them I was sleeping. Once the ward lights had been turned off, I sat on the cold linoleum floor next to the dirty washing trolley. This was the filthy place that I deserved. A number of nurses came and flashed their torches at me, but I remained silent and immoveable.

Wednesday 2 November 1994

I feel numb and overwhelmed by what has just happened. Jack's suggestion that we had some time alone together this evening was not so bad, until he suggested we go home. I could tell that having sex was important to Jack so I decided to manage the anxiety of being at home and 'making love' as best I could. I just could not reconcile the 'lovemaking' with the intensity of my earlier feelings. Sex was the last thing I needed or wanted.

I have felt in recent weeks, more than any other time, that Jack was going to give up on me. That he did not love me anymore. Tonight, he made a deep declaration of love. Dare I believe it? It is too much to assimilate. I need time to process it. How could it be that Jack could love me more now, than he ever has? Was he saying this just to have sex with me?

Persons who binge and purge usually make their depression worse,
but persons with anorexia are often able to suppress
that depression with their starving.
So when one of these persons is in treatment,
they're at a higher risk of suicide because that depression
is no longer masked by the eating disorder.
Dr. Lerner - Clinical Psychologist

Thursday 3 November 1994
I feel like a car that has run out of gas and has been left, abandoned. How can I feel this way when Jack has just declared his undying love for me? Why would I be in this state if that were true?

During my time with Chrissy today I told her the things Jack had said and done to me last night, and that it was hard to receive and accept them. There is something that I cannot reconcile.

The desire for death consumes me. In my mind I have a picture. There is a huge brick wall. On one side is 'life' - my family. I am desperately holding on to the other side of the unyielding and immovable wall with my face squashed up against it. I have no room to move because immediately behind me is a big black hole which I am teetering on the edge of. I am uncomfortable and scared. I do not know how much longer I can hold on. Why am I stuck in such a precarious position caught between an impenetrable wall and a black hole - unable to reach my family? It is too much for me.

I cannot get over the wall, but even if I could, I do not want to anymore. Any motivation and desire to try has gone. I am beaten! To allow myself to fall backwards into the hole would bring me release and relief but I would lose everything - my husband and family! Is this what I am afraid of? Is this fear holding all my illness in place?

Tuesday 8 November 1994

I lived yesterday in a peacefully defeated state, believing that the relinquishment of my life is both necessary and reasonable. This peace is very welcome.

A visit from Rebekah in the evening however, brought back the disturbing feelings. Having told her, quite unemotionally, of my resolve to die - she became determined and vigilant in her attempt to prevent this happening. Among other words she spoke, was a most passionate rendition of **Psalm130**:

Out of the depths I have cried to You, O Yehovah;
Lord, hear my voice!
Let Your ears be attentive
To the voice of my supplications.

If You, Yehovah, should mark iniquities,
O Lord, who could stand?
But there is forgiveness with You,
That You may be feared.
I wait for Yehovah, my soul waits,
And in His word I do hope.

My soul waits for the Lord
More than those who watch for the morning—
Yes, more than those who watch for the morning.
O Israel, hope in Yehovah;
For with Yehovah there is mercy,
And with Him is abundant redemption.
And He shall redeem Israel
From all his iniquities.

Before Rebekah left, this woman of faith told me that she would pray this prayer for me throughout the night. *"You'll need to pray hard!"* was my response to her. Unable to return to sleep at 2:00 am, I went to the ward lounge and sat watching the torrential rain flooding the courtyard. There had been no reprieve from the downpour of rain that flooded many parts of Wellington over the last couple of days. I had read Psalm 130 before going to bed. I dared God to intervene.

As I sat hearing the bellow of thunder, and watching the wind beating against the trees, the cracking of lightning, and the pelting horizontal rain, some changes within me were taking place. Should I feel frightened of what seems to be like nature out-of-control? Maybe its evidence of God's supreme control?

It is now 5:45 am. I have been watching this courtyard scene while enmeshed in my thoughts for nearly three hours. It is still raining and windy, but no longer tempestuous. My mood and thoughts are less tempestuous too.

How can it be and what has happened to make me now decide that I will live and that I am not going to be beaten? It has to be something supernatural that has happened within me. I do not know how, but I will make life work. Whatever it takes, I am going to get over that wall and away from that big black hole that until now has frightened, intimidated, immobilized and lured me. Could it be that Rebekah's prayers for me were answered?

The courtyard scene remains grey and uninviting, yet I allow myself to imagine it as a sunny, warm and welcoming place. I now accept to sit down between the brick wall and the black hole and rest. I must press the 'stop button' on my thinking now, as to think beyond this would be overwhelming.

2024 Spiritual Awakening:
Yehovah's Word is powerful! After all, Yehovah created the universe by His spoken Word! Rebekah had read Psalm 130 to me, she had prayed this prayer for me through the night hours, and I had read it before going to bed.

Yehovah says in Jeremiah 1:12 "*...I am ready to perform My word,*" and in Isaiah 55:11 Yehovah says, "*So shall My word be that goes forth from My mouth; It shall not return to Me void, but it shall accomplish what I please, and it shall prosper in the thing for which I sent it.*"

We can often underestimate the *very* great power and effect of saying Yehovah's very words back to Him, as we pray for ourselves and for others. Yehovah is waiting to answer prayers that line up with His Word, and every one of His words spoken out will accomplish His will and pleasure. That night, I received Yehovah's *forgiveness, mercy* and *abundant redemption*!

*****

Wednesday 9 November 1994

My appointment with Carmia gave me the opportunity to blurt out my tale. I then told her that I needed to know what my options were. Until the other night, it was as if I had accepted an inevitable defeat in a game of chess. I was convinced that I had no moves left. Yesterday I determined to find a move so as not to be defeated. As I do not have the necessary skill or insight myself, I decided to ask advice from another 'chess player.'

Carmia offered me two possible moves. One was to stay in the ward and look at making a discharge plan once she had returned from study leave on 21 November. I could have a gradual transition home, seeing Carmia daily. My other option was Ashburn Hall - a private psychiatric hospital in Dunedin. Carmia had spoken of this place before, but I had not seriously considered it.

My head had been whirling in confusion since talking with Carmia. I had asked her to start the application process for Dunedin. She thinks it is likely the CHE (Crown Health Enterprise) will provide the funding. My nurse told me I would me very fortunate if I did get the opportunity to go down to Ashburn Hall.

Questions and concerns flooded my head. What about Ruby? How would Jack cope? What was the hospital like? How could it help me? How long would I be there? Who do I know down there? It is such a long way away. So much expense and inconvenience to everyone. What if the DHB (District Health Board) will not pay? It is such a big decision to make.

Michelle sent me flowers from Christchurch today. These flowers, I have decided, are not going to be thrown away.

Saturday 12 November 1994
I go to Dunedin on Monday. Tomorrow is the last time I'll see Rebekah for while. She and Laurence have accepted an appointment in Hong Kong and will leave soon. Susan has been here to say goodbye. I wish she could come with me!

It's notoriously challenging to work with these patients,
even in a specialized setting with a lot of
[multi-disciplinary] support.
This is an incredibly challenging disorder.
Michael Rollin, MD - Psychiatrist
Eating Disorder Center of Denver

I left Ward 27 having received many kind and supporting words, hugs and a bottle of lavender oil from my nurse Rose. Lindsay took me to the airport. Other friends brought Ruby to the airport to say goodbye. Once I was on the plane and looking at Ruby's photographs, I experienced the full emotional impact of this Dunedin decision.

*****

CHAPTER 6

He Restores My Soul

Their soul abhorred all manner of food,
And they drew near to the gates of death.

Then they cried out to the Lord in their trouble,
And He saved them out of their distresses.

He sent His word and healed them,
And delivered them from their destructions.

Psalms 107:18-20

Ashburn Hall was a ninety-bed hospital which was founded in 1882. It accepted patients with a wide variety of psychiatric and emotional disorders and held to the concept of therapeutic community care. It was situated ten minutes from Dunedin's city center and surrounded by farmland. The grounds, which were extensive, were filled with shrubs, flower gardens and exotic trees which attracted a variety of native birds. There were ducks that waddled around the grounds in straight line formation. The rhododendrons and azaleas were a particular feature for me, as was the bush area that had a stream flowing through it. It was indeed a serene and inviting setting.

Alongside the main building was the recreation hall which was equipped for a variety of indoor sports and exercise. Next to this was an outdoor tennis court. The grounds also provided opportunity for other outdoor sport.

*****

She is kind and empathetic, deeply caring about how others feel and her own effect on their feelings. Her kindness and empathy work in his favor as well. When the abuser treats her poorly, she has already been trained to take on the responsibility for what he does.

Natalie Hoffman - Is It Me?

Monday 21 November 1994

It was a turbulent flight, and the wet Dunedin weather was less than welcoming. Bernadette and the girls (Dunedin friends) were there to meet me at the airport. Driving to Ashburn Hall seemed to take forever, as I tried unsuccessfully to quell my anxiety and apprehension.

After an initial interview, I was brought to the ward by Stacey, my 'buddy,' then got to meet a nurse called Monique. Throughout the assessment and interview with Monique, I sat looking out the window. It was grey, cold and raining.

I have a double bedroom all to myself. It is carpeted and heated. The other patients on this ward are young and appear to be sane. The floors are squeaky! My 'dangerous' belongings are being couriered down. Ward 27 staff did not trust me with them.

Tuesday 22 November 1993

I had a medical examination today. The doctor discovered the welts over my abdomen where I had been harming myself. I think she thought I had a strange skin disorder!

I had a session with Angela, my psychotherapist. To be in her room is like being in a tree-house. There were expansive windows around the room and treetops could be seen through each one of them. She seems nice enough, but having to develop a therapy relationship with someone new, makes me feel very alone and insecure. What if I do not do it right? What if she can't understand me? How long will it take before I find her helpful?

Wednesday 23 November 1994
More disturbing dreams.

Our daily ward meeting includes a round of feelings, where everyone says something of how they are feeling at the time. My word was 'hopeless.' Today I have felt lonely and unsupported. It is better to be known and disliked, than to be unknown. I wish I could be punched, kicked and hurt by everyone!

Monday 28 November 1994
I feel absolutely no benefit from sleep. When I do go to sleep, my dreams are disturbing and distressing for me. It is better not to let myself sleep. Last night was the worst dream ever. I woke up scared, confused, sweating profusely and hyperventilating. Jack, Ruby and I were to go away somewhere nice together. However, something happened so that Ruby went to Mary's which I knew to be a safe and secure place for her to be. Consequentl, she was not a part of the traumatic events that followed in the dream.

Instead of getting to the airport, Jack and I entered a house, was it our house? In each room I had to get rid of a supernatural presence. My body was extremely stressed and incapacitated. Jack was not helping me - he just watched - as I struggled with one demon after another! I had to evict each one. My weakened and almost ineffectual voice attempted to shout, *"Out, out!"* to each presence.

Horrible things were happening to me. My body was traumatized, confused, scared, panicked and fearful. The house had so many rooms, and so many doors to get them out. The voice had to be mine, though pathetic and weak. It was up to me to use what little strength I had to evict them. Why were they there, and why would they not leave willingly? Had Jack invited them? He did not seem surprised they were there.

I was partly awake each time I tried to say *"Out!"* and hoped someone in my real life would help me. They did not. This dream would not stop until I had gotten each demonic presence out of the front door. At this point, utterly exhausted, I knew I was in no fit state to go anywhere nice with Jack. I sobbed as I recounted the dream to the night nurse who jotted down my words. I also phoned Jack.

Tuesday 29 November 1994

More dreams. In one of them I was on a huge hovercraft. While at sea, everyone had to locate their individual lifeboats and venture off independently on the raging ocean. There was no emergency or damage to the hovercraft, this was just what everyone expected would happen at a certain stage of the voyage. Unlike everyone else who successfully launched and sailed their lifeboats from the hovercraft, my key to start the boat's engine would continually snap. It had to be repeatedly fixed. My dream ended with a broken key and me not having left the hovercraft.

Another dream was about having been weighed. I was commended for decreasing my weight to 99 kilograms (218 pounds)! I freak out at the thought of being weighed here on Mondays and Fridays.

I felt a lot of grief in my session with Angela today. I saw myself like a gift given to a child for Christmas. A spinning top all shiny and new that the child had really wanted. However, the novelty of the spinning top soon wore off for the child. After a few days the top was discarded and abandoned, left under the bed, outside or at the bottom of the toy box, getting little or no further attention. The spinning top created no more pleasure or joy.

*****

Evenings and weekends were free time. The rest of the week was quite structured and often intense. Within the weekly timetable were work groups, individual therapy, group therapy, ward activity, psychodrama, substance abuse group, eating disorder group, forum, sport and recreation, music and art therapy.

I was often up before 6:00 am each morning, 6:00 am was the time I met my mate - gym! We got to know each other really well over the time I was at Ashburn! Getting there at this time meant I would be guaranteed not to have my exercise program interrupted or delayed, which would have been extremely distressing for me. I vigorously worked the Exercycle, weights, punching bag and basketball net before doing my stretching exercises by the stream. Being able to get rid of some emotional energy at the punch-bag each morning helped me a lot - and I was obsessed with burning calories via exercise.

Dunedin was a long way away from the familiar, but I was fortunate to know a number of people down there. They not only visited and supported me, but they accommodated and cared for Jack and Ruby who flew down many weekends.

*****

Saturday 3 December 1994
My contracted 'talking time' with the Charge Nurse this morning took an unplanned direction. When we began, she felt it necessary to give some explanation to me as to what the present drama in the ward was about. A patient has hung herself and was found by two other patients. This has affected me profoundly. I questioned myself: Why her? Why not anyone else? It should have been me if anyone. What if it had been me? Such finality! So close, too close for comfort.

In consequence to this new source of emotional turmoil, I handed over to the Charge Nurse quite a reasonable number of my hoarded anti-depressants that I had not been taking. I was keeping them as a back-up option, just in case this place cannot help me. I cannot trust myself after knowing of this woman's death.

It seems so disrespectful to me that when someone dies, life just continues on as normal as if nothing has ever happened. Surely the world should stop! What right have I to have a nice bedroom, a beautiful daughter, a new sweater in light of this woman's death?

Sunday 4 December 1994
I panicked this morning as the gym was all locked up, and I had limited time before Jack and Ruby arrived.

This morning Ruby, Jack and I decided to do something quite unusual. We went to a church service! The only reason for this strange and bizarre behavior was that my 'buddy' from the ward was involved in a young people's Christmas musical that she had invited us to. As we entered the Mosgiel Presbyterian Church, I was quite moved by the warmth, life and welcome I experienced. I was further surprised as the words of the pastor's opening prayer included, *"Some people here today do not know how to live, what to do, or what to believe..."* I had not ever heard these accepting, sensitive, perceptive, comforting and soothing words in a church before!

Monday 5 December 1994
It was all the 'F' words in the 'feelings round' for me today. Frantic, fatigued, fearful and fragile.

I have a friend here called Catherine. To know her is to love her. Already we have shared many a happy and despairing moment together. I am glad of her friendship, and our badminton games.

Friday 9 December 1994
Many nights I am up till 1, 2 or 3:00 am, painting paper, making cards or photo-frames, or doing my cut-and-salvage with the <u>hundreds</u> of magazines. This magazine and junk mail thing is no joke! As much as I want Priscilla and Gillian to keep bringing magazines in for me, and am pleased that this place has huge stashes of them, this obsession and compulsion is wearing me out. I want it to stop.

Saturday 10 December 1994
Yesterday I saw some beautiful flowers being delivered to reception. I thought, *what a lucky person to be receiving them.* A few minutes later they were brought down to my room! They were from Gwen, Jack's aunt.

Monday 12 December 1994
Today was a significant day. While in town with Jack and Ruby, I bought a dress. This is the first I will have worn for four years. This is a transition time - I am taking off my 'grave clothes' (my gothic black).

Tuesday 20 December 1994
Susan writes and tells me that she sees me as a sailboat. The waters I sail on are sometimes smooth, peaceful and clear. Other times rough and tempestuous. I am often in dock for repair work, but in time I will fulfill my destiny! A ship in the harbor is safe, but that is not what ships are built for.

Michelle told me on the telephone the other day, that she sees me as a dancer - strong and graceful - but wearing a heavy boot on one foot. This limits and prevents me from fully experiencing and displaying the freedom and beauty that one day will be mine.

Thursday 22 December 1994
Food is occupying my mind full-time. I noticed there were biscuits left out in the kitchen last night and it put me at risk. Having eaten two, I forced myself outside to use the cell-phone instead of giving in to the temptation to binge.

Friday 23 December 1994
I was weighed this morning. I made a decision to be firmer with myself but ate a scone for morning tea. The desire to reverse it was strong, but I found two other patients and talked it through with them. The rejection of food is symbolic of rejecting anything nice or good.

Sunday 25 December 1994
Yesterday when Jack's father picked me up, he asked me how I felt about going to Christchurch. I told him that the whole food issue was overwhelming. His response was, *"well in reality, we only spend approximately an hour and a half eating each day, so..."* If only my wild, wayward, tormenting and destructive food thoughts could be nicely contained to a daily one and a half hours.

Wednesday 28 December 1994
Apart from the times and moments of pleasure with Ruby - Christmas was again an experience I would rather forget. I have come back to Ashburn with a desperate inner cry to be saved from myself.

While in Christchurch, my lack of faith and trust in myself grew more severe the longer I was there. Not only was I overwhelmed and indecisive about food, but other things as well. I have been angry and agitated with myself, eating so much. Being back at Ashburn will bring some boundaries again. Is this just wishful thinking. There is no respite from this food temptation until after New Year!

Although there is a measure of relief about being back here at Ashburn, the source of my distress has come back with me and will forever be with me because it is me!

Monday 2 January 1995
This morning Monique asked me why I had not fronted up for my last couple of weigh-ins. I thought she was not only disappointed with me, but also angry. I have talked with her about this just now. She asked me why I have always equated disappointment with anger. It is true, if anyone is ever disappointed with me, I have thought they were also angry with me. If I disappoint myself, I am also angry with myself.

Thursday 5 January 1995
Today in group therapy I was an emotional wreck. It was the longest hour of group ever. I desperately wanted to escape as my emotions were so difficult to contain. The focus eventually was on me. It was not for the lack of wanting to share, but I just could not. It was too big, too much, and no words. What was it?

FAT FAT FAT

These overwhelming *fat attacks* and feelings of self-disgust, what are they really about? I must determine the real issues at stake.

Friday 6 January 1995
Sarah tried to hang herself the other night. Since then a special nurse has been constantly at her bedside. She does not want life. I have sat with Sarah for an hour and a half today while a special nurse was being organized. As well as massaging her hands, I wrote her this poem:

As I sit at your side
Aware of your pain and despair
Your hopelessness and blackness
What can I say or do to ease your troubled
and despondent spirit?

A woman of beauty and grace
Yet you do not perceive this.
A woman of utmost value and worth
Yet you do not perceive this.
A woman of destiny and potential
Yet you do not perceive this.

My heart hurts to know that blindness to
these things robs you of all
Life, Happiness and Peace.

"Death" screams out at me from you and I scream back,
"Life, Life, Life."

The green pine needles you so tentatively perch on
beside the big, black, alluring hole are of little comfort
Yet for those of us who refuse to let you fall,
they are a symbol of the forest that lies beyond your
insurmountable and unyielding black wall.

The forest waits longingly for you to experience its
beauty, refreshment and strength.

I will not lose hope for you, Sarah my friend.

Sunday 8 January 1995
Banana cake was brought into the ward today. My mouth made a verbal decline as a piece was offered me, but my mind said *"yes."* I later stole a piece. It was nice to eat but wrong to keep. It was so bad because it tasted so good.

Catherine and I have a secret code word that we say to each other if we are in food conflict and need support from the other - *badminton*. But it is usually said, *"BADMINTON!"* because of the inner turmoil or desperation we are feeling.

Monday 9 January 1995
The weekend has been very raging and tempestuous on the ward. Self-harming, threats and attempts of suicide, heightened emotions, and neediness. Christmas and New Year has been an extremely stressful time for most people here.

Tuesday 17 January 1995
We got back to Dunedin yesterday. As Jack and Ruby will not be able to come down again - this is the last time I will see them here. Perhaps it will be possible for me to make a weekend trip home in February.

Thursday 19 January 1995
Why is it that I am unable to establish and maintain eye contact in a therapy session? I do not feel like an okay person. I do not feel deserving of their time, of imposing on people's time. To make eye contact would be to assume that I am worthy of time, and that it is reasonable for me to have help and support.

I feel sad and homesick. I have spent most of the day in my room. I did not even attend ward meeting or forum. I have decided that I will go home 27th of January. This is very soon, but to my grieving and homesick state it is not soon enough. I am not sure if this non-negotiable decision is right.

Friday 20 January 1995

The Church

> *If this is not a place where tears are understood, then where shall I go to cry? I do not need another place for trying to impress you with just how good and virtuous I am. No, no, no. I do not need another place for always being on top of things. Everybody knows that it is a sham. I do not need another place for always wearing smiles - even when it is not the way I feel. I do not need another place to mouth the same old platitudes. Everyone knows it is not real.*

So if this is not a place where my questions can be asked, then where shall I go to seek? And if this is not a place where my heart-cry can be heard, where, tell me where, shall I go to speak? So if this is not a place where tears are understood, where shall I go? Where shall I go to cry?

- Anonymous

Sunday 22 January 1995
I rang our friend Rob last night as the guilt and confusion I had about my parents being the source of my illness caused me great distress. I talked and cried with him for ages. He was finally able to ground me. He also encouraged me to write my parents a letter.

Dear Mum and Dad,

I write to tell you of my intention of returning to Wellington on 27 January. However, there is also something more I would wish to say.

I do realize that the difficulties I have experienced in these recent years, and of course even now, have also resulted in difficult times for you. I am really not sure what to say to you, other than to let you know I have never set out to hurt you. Things may seem out of kilter at present, but I do not think it will be like this forever. You might also in time come to realize why certain things have had to be.

Cate

Monday 23 January 1995
It is only Monday and already I am packing and clearing my walls.

In art therapy today we were asked to paint or draw a picture using appropriate colors that expressed our feelings. I painted the entire paper bright orange and then splattered it with various other bright colors. This expressed and encapsulated my anticipation of going home. The excitement of being with Ruby again. It has been four months since we visited the zoo, library, and the pools.

Ashburn Hall obliged my request to read my clinic files. At admission my diagnosis was seen as Anorexia Nervosa. The psychiatrist further wrote: ***"Presumably her eating disorder and these conflicts have their origins in her early relationship with her mother.*** *She is a very good candidate for psychotherapy, especially within the therapeutic community."*

Thursday 26 January 1995
My time with Angela this morning was the least satisfying and most distressing session I've had with her. Obviously, I had not made my intentions of leaving clear to her.

Although she was aware that I planned to leave tomorrow, I had not told her Jack wished to have my bed saved for me for a week in case I needed to return. I wonder why Jack made this request. Does Jack want me to remain in the psych ward? Angela appeared stressed because this arrangement meant that the discharge letter she had written was now inappropriate. So, officially, I am only on leave due to Jack's request.

Friday 27 January 1995 - My birthday!
As I was up at 3:45 am in readiness for my afternoon flight, the night nurse came into my room and wished me a happy birthday. The day of my departure was grey and wet as it had been the day I arrived. Many kind words were expressed to me in the ward meeting. Angela said that she regrets our work together cannot continue and that she wished she could be my real therapist instead of the foster role she fulfilled. It is also her birthday today. I want to go home but I do not want to leave.

While there are some dire statistics related to eating disorders and suicide rates, there are also plenty of stories of hope. There are people who recover and who go on to live full lives. The stakes are high with eating disorders in that things tend to either go really well or really wrong, and there's not a lot in between the two extremes.

Michael Rollin, MD

Eating Disorder Center of Denver

Wednesday 1 February 1995

After four months, it is really good to be home again. We have been going through each room of the house sorting, sifting, assimilating and abandoning. Our decision has been to ruthlessly part with the old, so is to make room for the new. We have gathered a lot since our last sorting episode, not the least of which is in Ruby's bedroom. She has accumulated an enormous amount in her last four months of growing and living.

I have been bought some new clothes to replace my grave clothes. No skirts or dresses. I doubt that I will ever be much of a skirt and dress wearer again. My old black boots are gone. My black trousers have been ripped up with great delight!

Thursday 2 February 1995

Prior to my time at Ashburn Hall, life for me was neither manageable or desirable. I had no fight or drive. The change brought with it inner strength, a willingness and desire to live. In retrospect, I think the first turning point in ward 27 gave me feelings of wanting life, but I was without the skills to make it happen.

2024 Spiritual Awakening: Remember how Judah and his household (Joseph's family) were living in Canaan when severe famine came? And how Yehovah had positioned Joseph in Egypt, through trial and tribulation, to be the answer to their needs? See Genesis 39 - 45.

Well… faced with starvation, Joseph's family would have died, except that Joseph brought them out of Canaan, and with Pharaoh's permission, gave them the fertile land of Goshen in Egypt, where

Jacob and his son's families lived and thrived. It was a place free from the distress they had previously experienced in Canaan, where they faced the prospect of starvation and death.

The families of Jacob lived in Goshen until Joseph and the Pharaoh of that time eventually died. The new Pharaoh of Egypt did not remember Joseph, or respect Joseph's God, as his predecessor had. This new Pharaoh's rule over the Israelites was brutal. Goshen, the place that had once been a place of help and rescue for the children of Israel, became a place of cruelty, that held the Israelites in bondage and slavery to Pharaoh.

Strangely, I see a curious parallel in my life to Joseph's family, as I look back to Ashburn Hall. I see how Ashburn Hall had been a place of rescue and help for those like me distressed with anorexia, as Egypt had been a place of help and rescue to Jacob's household when facing starvation through famine. Some years later I was to again be admitted to Ashburn, now called *Ashburn Clinic,* and under very different staffing. It was no longer a place of help and rescue, but had become a place of cruelty, and brutal treatment of patients. I will relate more in chapter ten, 'The Pit.'

Monday 6 February 1995
Today we have been married seven years (going on seventy). Since my marriage began, I have been on a roller coaster. I go from bad to worse, dragging myself up the rope to sanity again - then repeat the cycle! Why is it getting harder each time to pull myself back to sanity? What does that say about me and my situation? My marriage?

2024 Looking Back: I have two answers to these questions of mine. Firstly, the imbalance of power in our marriage, had an eroding effect on me and on my ability to be well and stay well. It was the **imbalance of power**, coercion and control that created the emotional abuse in our marriage. Secondly, I came to see that Jack could not tolerate me being well and strong - which would have been an **imbalance of power**. Jack could not manage that amount of insecurity.

Wednesday 8 February 1995
Ruby is two years old today.

Jack does not feel he is as helpful to me as people like Rebekah and Rose are. In fact, he wonders if he is helpful to me at all. I realized while talking about this with Carmia, that I do not encourage him with positive feed-back. There is definitely a level of support and understanding he cannot give.

I need to learn how to nurture my soul. The disturbing feelings I have of my heart being cold, hard, unreachable and encrusted may well be indicators of this need. Now, I am having to start from the beginning again. It is as if I threw out the baby with the bath water. The bath symbolizing my soul. Now I have my bath (soul) back, but I am not sure about the baby (my faith) and the water (my beliefs). But it is a start.

Thursday 9 February 1995
Is there anything strong, lasting, and real about church culture? Is there anything more than spiritual sentimentality? It is so taunting and illusive to me. If there is a God who can give my life meaning, foundation and substance, then let me know Him. My own experience, and what I see in others, sometimes tells me there isn't. However, I have a need within me to prove this wrong.

Tuesday 14 February 1995
On Sunday morning I went to see nurse Rose at the psychiatric unit for some support. I told her that I am not always able to articulate my feelings in an instant as Jack wants me to. I recognize that Jack's need to identify what is happening is his way of attempting to gain control over an 'out of control' situation. Rose suggests that I shouldn't allow Jack's need for control to discredit my feelings. I also told Rose that my feelings towards Jack were not what I'd like them to be. Often, I wonder if I love him at all! Maybe I'm grieving the loss of Jack not being what I had always believed him to be.

Wednesday 15 February 1995
I am now beginning to experience grief and loss about the church. The fear and anger I have towards the church is part of the grieving

process, I think. We grieve any loss, and the church is a loss for me. It is not what I once believed it to be. It has not met my needs. I have felt disappointed, hurt and let down.

I cannot eradicate the church from my life, like drugs or alcohol. I believe in God, and the church is God's institution even though it so often misrepresents Him. I have to grieve the loss of perfection while still accepting the positive part that remains.

Spirituality may include the
organized form of the Church,
but I am mighty sure that it must transcend it!

What can dissipate my shame? Ultimately God I suppose. Perhaps this toxic shame has already started to dissipate.

2024 Spiritual Awakening:
Shame is an outright attack of Satan. **Truth dissipates shame.**

Wednesday 12 April 1995
My escape plan for difficult or undermining situations has always been to run or hide. Instead of doing this I need to cut off my escape routes and face the situation. In talking with Carmia about one distressing dream I had while at Ashburn Hall, she asked me to assume the role of the intimidator. She asked, *"What was my name? What did I look like? What did I do?"*

"I will not tell you my name or disclose my appearance. What I do, is make Cate fearful. I drain her of every ounce of energy. I weaken her and make her feel helpless and alone. I am resistant, stubborn and aggressive. I will go, but it will take every bit of Cate's energy and desire to evict me. Of course the back door is always an option for my sneaky return!"

"Does Cate want you to go?" "Yes."

In my dream, I spoke in an extremely weakened state and voice, *"out"* through each room of house. Room after endless room, till the presence was out the front door. I could not identify this 'presence' as a person, but rather as an evil influence or spiritual presence, a demon perhaps. Male, I think. Familiar, I think.

*****

Friday 14 April 1995

Good Friday. Another walk up Melrose Hill and beyond. I spoke with God about how I feel when I give a gift to someone and it's unappreciated, especially when the gift is something that I have made. The recipient does not seem to appreciate the thought, time and effort that's gone into it. Little response or acknowledgment is made. It is not talked about or shared with others. You never see it displayed or used. What has become of it? Did it even get a second look before being discarded? Maybe they did not understand its worth.

But there are other people who will receive a gift you give them and have a great response. They recognize the thought, time and effort. They will sometimes even share the gift with others.

And so, on this Good Friday, I reflect on God's gift to me. Jesus. A gift that is the most precious and costly. What response will I make to God? I expressed a desire to God for Him to help me understand His gift - the significance to me, the value and cost, how I could find pleasure and excitement in it, and so want to enthusiastically share it with others. To recognize the "pearl" as being of "great price!"

Tuesday 18 April 1995

I feel like an overworked washing machine that is rapidly wearing out and depreciating. Every cycle is on heavy-duty and as soon as the washing cycle is finished, another load that has been waiting is immediately shoved in. The machine is continually working with no respite. It does not sit nice and tidy and clean for a while, used only just once a week. It has become shabby and dirty. This is the sort of machine that soon gets trashed and traded or discarded.

Wednesday 19 April 1995
Is the relationship I have had with my parents really as bad as I make out?

Wednesday 26 April 1995
I was suddenly debilitated by my emotions last night. Jack was frustrated and angry with the situation, yet it felt as if his responses were all directed at me. I felt shattered when I arrived at the hospital for my appointment this morning.

I often have an overwhelming desire to escape, die or for the end of the world to come, so as not to feel continuing pain and loss, failure and shame. There is no security, consistency or surety in life.

Monday 1 May 1995
Although I still have the non-coping feelings today, they are not overwhelming me as they did yesterday. Things have changed in me since six months ago. These feelings do not lead me into self-destructive behavior.

2024 Looking Back:

But he who is joined to Adonai (the Lord) is one spirit with Him.
1 Corinthians 6:17

I had come up from the abyss. I am in a much better place for sure. During those months at Ashburn Hall, I felt like I had found my soul again. I went from being incapacitated to deciding to write this book. I had opened a door. I had support and was eager to get back to my daughter Ruby.

She is generous—giving more than she
takes and doing it with joy.
Because she is generous, she pours all her resources
into the marriage, whatever they may be,
believing she is investing in the most worthwhile
relationship God has ordained for her.
Natalie Hoffman - Is It Me?

CHAPTER 7

House On The Rock

So it shall be, when Yehovah your God brings you into the land...
to give you large and beautiful cities which you did not build,
and houses full of all good things...
Deuteronomy 6:10-11

Saturday 13 May 1995
Prior to my marriage in 1989, I had a 'house' that looked fine. By 1991 my 'house' had fallen to the ground. The foundations lay in ruins. Now, four years since the demolition work began, I see myself as having a new foundation laid. Nothing beyond the foundation work has yet been done. The work site is very open, vulnerable and exposed, with nothing private or hidden. I am not sure what the end result will be like, the plans are still in in the hands of God - the Architect.

Tuesday 16 May 1995
I have high hopes about what my 'house' will be like. The enormity of the task, however - keeps me from thinking beyond the foundation. I do not know where to go from here.

Yeshua said -

Therefore whoever hears these sayings of Mine, and does them,
I will liken him to a wise man who built his house on the rock:
and the rain descended, the floods came,
and the winds blew and beat on that house;
and it did not fall, for it was founded on the rock.
But everyone who hears these sayings of Mine, and does not do them,
will be like a foolish man who built his house on the sand:

and the rain descended, the floods came,
and the winds blew and beat on that house; and it fell.
And great was its fall.
Matthew 7:24-27

*****

Wednesday 24 May 1995
I saw Chrissy today. At one point in the session I felt overwhelming sadness and shame. I also felt apologetic for my existence. When Chrissy asked me why, I said I didn't know. I just did. Chrissy doesn't think we just feel these things without a cause. Rather, they are messages we have received from others. Chrissy tried to help me uncover what happened in my childhood to cause these feelings.

*****

2024 Looking Back:
Chrissy wrongly assumed that my feelings had originated from childhood experiences. I still did not recognize that my feelings were a result of emotional and sexual abuse in my marriage. Women often do not reveal sexual abuse in marriage - not even in counseling. Shame is a contributing factor to this, but victims also experience confusion about what is happening to them. Women may feel defiled but think it is unreasonable for them to feel this way. **And so it was for me when I became aware of Jack's desire for pornography.**

Women may not recognize sexual abuse in their marriage
for several reasons: Fear of retaliation or violence,
Fear of being judged or blamed, Fear of being abandoned or
rejected, Fear of being labeled as "crazy" or "overly sensitive,"
Lack of knowledge about what constitutes sexual abuse,
Feeling trapped or stuck in the relationship.
Focus on the Family

The first I knew of Jack's issue with pornography was when he wanted me to watch pornography with him on a purchased television channel. As with his other sexually deviant fetishes, he normalized this to me. He would say things like, *"This is fine. We're married so it can't be wrong."* Or, *"This will help make our sex better!"* Or *"This is what our relationship needs."* When I objected, Jack would say I was hung-up and not free enough to have good marital sex - I was denying him. I remember watching something pornographic with him under duress. It was sickening to me!

I told Jack I was never going to do that again! He did not ask me to watch anything like this with him again but he continued to use pornography, as I found out later. The other fetishes also continued to increase year after year - I had tried to draw a line. To some readers this may not be a big deal - but sexual pornography and other fetishes are ungodly and deeply offensive to me.

I felt deeply scandalized and wounded by being coerced to do these things. I did not understand why Jack would condone this - he was a minister! Living with all this sexual deviancy being forced on me, crashed my sense of morality. My moral compass was being destroyed but this objectification and control. Step by step Jack dragged me deeper and deeper into the morass of sexual perversion. I was purposely deceived. With these constant indecent demands upon me, my belief in what was right and wrong, slipped from my grasp. Once Jack had habituated me to a certain level of indecency, he would up the ante.

I would later learn that the first step in abuse or terrorism is to turn the person into a thing - an object, a function - not a person.

...he is in her head telling her it's all her fault.
She believes this is true—
that if she would have tried harder or been different
or responded differently, she could have made things better.
Natalie Hoffman - Is It Me?

Friday 26 May 1995

Today was my first session back with Carmia. I don't feel ready for another transition, but then I never do. There is always an enormous chasm to be leapt before I can feel known and secure again. The effort often seems too much - beyond me. My silence is my grief. I quite purposely dropped my cup of hot water on the floor. I was upset with myself for this grief.

Chrissy had obviously had a debrief with Carmia. Chrissy must have said to Carmia that I was without purpose in my life. This was true enough, but for Carmia to interpret this as meaning that my life was empty, was quite incorrect! At this suggestion I replied, *"No, no, no. It is too full. I wish I could be emptied of all the thoughts, feelings, expectations, sadness, and heaviness."*

I feel a continual sense of heaviness about living. I cannot imagine what it must be like to wake up in the morning and feel charged up and ready for the day ahead, or to think *"ah... life is good."* I am surprised that others cannot see this heavy weight that persistently sits on my shoulders. Is it not visible?

Saturday 27 May 1995

Depression and anxiety must be causing this horrible heaviness. Is it because I fear losing the precious things of life? Anything can be taken away in an instant of time without warning? The worst thing that could happen to me, would be to lose Ruby, or Jack. That is unthinkable to me. I cannot face it.

Real loss and the threat of loss makes life too painful for me much of the time, and so I want to hide, escape or cop-out. Certainly I try to block-out the losses, hurts and pain of others so as not to be overwhelmed by them. Perhaps these responses are because of my vulnerability. The fact is that I am still standing on a very open and exposed foundation that offers no protection, security or refuge from life's onslaughts.

I have made SOS telephone calls to both Carmia and Chrissy at various times when feeling alone or when in an overwhelmed or incapacitated state. At the time I can't tell them specifically how they can help me. I don't even know what to say.

2024 Looking Back:
My relationship with Jack created a lot of confusion for me. The landscape was always moving to suit Jack's need for power and control. I came to realize that I was not always living in my reality but in Jack's reality, because he had a need for me to think like he did. Anything less than that was intolerable. This was just as much the case with Jack's sexual abuse.

Sexual abuse has devastating impacts on a person,
and those impacts compound when the
abuse occurs in a marriage.
Two of those impacts — faith struggles and shame —
leave a victim confused and often silent.
Focus on the Family

Sexual abuse resulted in me feeling alone and depressed, like when Jack had me role-play being a prostitute called "Candy."

My Name is "Candy"

To the erotic lingerie that had started Jack's sexual abuse by coercion, were added sex toys and other clothing items that he selected and purchased for me to wear for him. There was even a slutty lace-up corset with matching underwear. Jack coerced me to act as his prostitute with the name "Candy." When I was dressed up in nothing but black underwear, fishnet stockings, high black boots, and a long black tailored coat - he had me go out the back door of our house and then go to the front door of our house. There I would knock on the door and Jack would open it and greet me, before escorting me into our bedroom. I was addressed as *"Candy"* throughout the sexual encounter.

I definitely did not want to do this. I felt intensely objectified by these and many other sexual experiences with Jack. I was no longer Cate, Jack's wife. I was Candy the prostitute who was sexually servicing Jack to fulfill his fantasies. This was another blow to my personhood, to my self-esteem. I was no longer a wife. I was a thing to be used. It was degrading. I felt numb, depressed and shamed.

I was told - and believed - that sex was the only thing I had to offer Jack. I was after all, not a well and functioning equal in our marriage. We were not sharing life interdependently and mutually edifying each other in our roles as husband and wife. I was sick and needy and required so much from Jack. He was my savior. This was the least I could do to pay him back for saving me! My sense of my own value as a wife and woman took a nose-dive. My depression deepened.

Sexual coercion is confusing, because if the wife acquiesces, she believes that she's agreed to have sex. It's then difficult for her to be clear about what has happened to her.
Focus on the Family

*****

Thursday 1 June 1995
Until my marriage, the outside of me was still intact and complete looking. Now, I am on the operating table with a great incision down the front of me - open and vulnerable - not in a state to cope and interact with life as other well people would.

There are many times that I wish I could talk with others without being seen. A desire to be invisible. My present overwhelming 'fat' feelings are the reason. It is extremely difficult to face people, and it is a real effort to interact. I cannot make eye contact. I can hardly handle seeing myself - let alone others seeing me.

Friday 23 June 1995

We are at Jack's parents. I have had my first reversing slip since Ashburn Hall. I had eaten ice-cream, then chocolate. Jack's father forced me to confess I had eaten as much chocolate as everyone else! It was all too much!

Saturday 1 July 1995

Although I still feel like a hopeless reject, I know that I am not. So why do I still identify myself as an old car with a broken-own engine, missing wheels, a damaged and unsightly body?

2024 Looking Back:

While I was going through the valley of the shadow of death, Satan tried in every way he could to make me give up, quit and die. He was close to succeeding in his efforts to destroy my life many times. In these times Satan would try to convince me that:

Yehovah did not care about me or love me. My life was not worth anything - so not worth saving. Yehovah had forsaken me in my darkness, pain and suffering because I was too wretched to be forgiven. Yehovah was powerless to rescue me as I had gone too far. I was all alone. Change was not possible - so there was no way out for me other than death!

In my darkest times, I often believed Satan! As best as I could, I held on to Yehovah, but when I could not, Yehovah held onto me! I came to see how Satan was trying to destroy me. Yehovah allowed these times to strengthen me. Yehovah had not put me in these dire circumstances. Yehovah was getting me through all of this crisis to the way out.

Thankfully I had a friend, Mary, to help me with Ruby throughout this difficult time.

*****

....she has no desire to betray or expose her partner.
Her heart is for him. Her motive is to help him so they can
have an intimate relationship that is mutually satisfying.
Against all the evidence to the contrary,
she continues to believe this is possible,
and her first attempts at getting help are for the sole
and desperate purpose of achieving this end.
However, most Churches and Bible counselors
won't be able to understand her or her problem.
The voice of her abuser is in their head, too.
In fact, they feed off one another and abuse the woman together.
Natalie Hoffman - Is It Me?

*****

Friday 7 July 1995
My self-destructive way of thinking continually attempts to overthrow the new me. How long will this dichotomy of thought and feeling prevail? Much of the time I feel as if I have a split personality! I can think two opposing thoughts and don't know which to believe. My mind is so confused.

Sunday 16 July 1995
While in session with Carmia today I felt a deep sadness. Carmia thinks I feel sadness to stop myself feeling angry. What am I angry about, Jack, my parents, myself?

Take the rope
from my throat that I may sing
my song...
Whakatohea chief Mokomoko, 1866 New Zealand

Thursday 20 July 1995
I imagine this scenario... a woman is married to an alcoholic and abusive partner for many years. There comes a day when she can no longer remain in a relationship that is destroying her. For her own survival, she makes the decision to leave him.

Why am I imagining this? Jack is not alcoholic. Am I questioning whether I can stay in a relationship with him? Is our relationship destroying me? I cannot imagine leaving him - but, in fact, that is exactly what I am imagining! It is a supremely scary thought!

2024 Looking Back:
Jack regularly had a thing for me performing oral sex on him. Something I desperately hated doing. Even now, just to mention it, fills me fear and a traumatic recall to throw up. I was also sodomized regularly by Jack. Why would anyone want to do that to a woman? For all of these unwanted sexual acts, Jack coerced me, saying it was what sexually healthy couples did. I would ask him how he knew this, and he would tell me he had read it.

Men sexually abuse their wives by coercing, forcing
or manipulating partners into sexual behaviors that they
are not comfortable with or have previously said "no" to.
Focus on the Family

Monday 24 July 1995
It seems to me that my emotional pantry has been mixed up. Fear has been in the 'FAT' container. Shame has been in the 'Abuse' container. Anger has been in the 'Sadness' container. Abandonment has been in the 'Lonely' container.

Feelings of shame, abandonment, fear, rejection and unimportance are like thick, sticky, messy, molasses that has become impossible to wade through.

Monday 31 July 1995

Identifying, facing and feeling the fears I have is a hard thing to do. I am no longer just saying, *"I am fat."* I am expressing the fears and pain specifically when I say things like, *"I fear loss. I fear being abandoned. I fear losing my husband, my family."* Yet I cannot, or perhaps will not, admit to myself or others the real source of my anger. Am I searching for the root of my problem in the wrong place? Why is it always my parents who are blamed?

Carmia has caused me to consider a change. Being able to move with heavy feelings is better than being stuck with heavy feelings, as was the case for me until not too long ago. It takes so much effort to function and manage my life, but life *is* better. But what does this change mean for me? What part do I have in my family?

The aim of therapy, Carmia tells me, is to sort the thinking, feelings and old messages, many of which were not helpful, and to re-write my life story. Re-writing my story allows me to be more truthful, free and gentle with myself.

2024 Spiritual Awakening:

Trust in Him at all times, you people;
Pour out your heart before Him;
God is a refuge for us. Selah
Psalm 62:8

I did a lot of pouring out my heart to therapists, as one might pour water out of a pitcher and into a glass. However, I did a poor job of p*ouring out my heart to Yehovah* - throughout my marriage to Jack.

The original Hebrew meaning of *pouring out* means to express without restraint, and is an act of trusting Yehovah. Pouring out our hearts to Yehovah, is saying, *"I am pouring out my heart to You Father, because I need You. I am relying on You to help me through this situation. I am desperate for Your help. You are my only hope."*

Hannah modeled this to us in 1 Samuel 1-2. She brought the full weight of her grief, sadness, disappointment, hurt and every other emotion to Yehovah, knowing that He was the only One truly strong enough to handle the weight of all her emotions.

Pouring out our hearts,
is an act of trusting Yehovah.

While there was value for me in pouring out my heart to mental health professionals, I realize now that Yehovah was grieved that I did not pour out my heart to Him. I had more trust in people, including Jack, than I did in my loving Creator. Again, I am *so* sorry Abba!

My Abba-Yehovah was the best and most important One to pour out my heart to. And prayer would have changed me, the pray-er, even before it changed the circumstances I was in.

*****

Wednesday 9 August 1995
I have started writing a book. Yesterday afternoon I finished another chapter. I had spent a lot of time on it, and although I knew it needed more work, I thought it was good in its raw state.

I printed it out for Jack to read. He gave me little response or feed-back. To me, this was a sure sign that my writing was bad. I became wrought with emotion. I later realized that these emotions were shame and fear, yet at the time they were being camouflaged by my self-hatred and disgust. All I wanted was to rip up the chapter, block it out, and pretend it had never existed. I was angry with myself for having let Jack read something so stupid, unintelligent and meaningless. All this anguish was because Jack did not respond.

I have been seeking Jack's approval, and blessing, on each chapter. This time I did not receive it - I was devastated! I could not possibly publish something Jack didn't approve of! As I lay on the floor sobbing and non-responsive, Jack got into his, 'let me talk some sense into you mode.' This was code for a long criticism dump upon me ending with "get a grip." He was wanting to bring control to a seemingly out-of-control situation. He told me that we were both able to deal with the situation more maturely. What he meant, was that I was being immature! He went on to say that I was being stubborn and resistant.

Once Ruby was in bed, Jack sat down beside me on the hall floor to re-read my chapter. This was too much for me! I got up and stood at the far end of the hall, facing the corner in the dark, and sobbing into my hands. I was crying my 'headache cry.' I cried intensely until I had a headache. This did not help Jack's response.

It was only as I stood there that I identified the feelings of shame and fear which had overwhelmed and engulfed me. I had desperately been trying to work it out all along, even though Jack thought otherwise. Jack followed me into the bedroom as I crawled into bed. Only then could I start to respond to him and tell him what was happening.

I realized that although he was right when he had said I was acting in bad old ways, it was actually appropriate and necessary for me. The behavior was part of the process I had to go through, as long as I had the permission to do so. I had to go through the pseudo issue with its associated emotions in order to discover the real issue and associated emotions. The surface issue was the book chapter with the anger and self-hatred. The underlying issue was my struggle with Jack over the value of my efforts.

Jack told me when I lay face down on the floor, he was left to stand by confused and unable to help. I told him that he was not a bystander at all. That although this was his perception, my reality was that he had me pinned to the ground as he stood with his foot on my back.

His verbal onslaught that attempted to bring control and rationality to the situation, prevented me from understanding and resolving the situation for myself. These differing perceptions have frequently happened over the past years. Jack blamed them on me, my therapists blamed them on my parents - I am beginning to see how it all centers around Jack. Why does everything I write have to be approved by Jack anyway?

Fear constantly drives the limbic part of my brain. Not to have Jack's approval is bad. It is anguish! Worse is to write something Jack absolutely does not like! That sends me into a tearful breakdown where I feel stupid and inconsequential. The worst is to anger Jack so completely that I could be abandoned. This is my greatest fear.

A very similar thing had happened for Ruby in tandem with me. Not too unlike other nights recently, she would not go to the toilet, brush her teeth, get her pajamas on or stay in bed. Jack was getting cross with her, and she was getting even more upset and unobliging. In the later part of the evening, she had not even been using words to communicate to us, but rather she used her behavior to express her frustration and annoyance with us. We could not understand what it was she was needing or wanting from us. This of course only served to compound my distress, no doubt as mine had compounded hers.

Jack stopped talking at me so he could spend some time talking with Ruby once she was in bed. He finally got to know what was really bothering Ruby. Her 'acting out' behavior, was because she wanted

Jack or I to stay with her in her bedroom. She was scared of the tiger from *Jungle Book* coming to get her.

Just as it was quite inappropriate, and unhelpful for Jack to tell me I was being stubborn and resistant when I was experiencing acute shame and fear, it was also inappropriate and unhelpful for us to be cross with Ruby for her supposed stubbornness and resistance, when she was in fact fearful.

Friday 11 August 1995

In all my dreams, I am surrounded by lots of people. I am on the outside of a group in which I once belonged - family, church, friends, nursing colleagues. In my dreams I am attempting to find a different way of getting back into the group without compromising my autonomy and true self. I am scared of becoming merged and lost again. If I am to be a part of these groups again, my self must remain clearly defined.

Wednesday 16 August 1995

Dramatic changes are happening so fast. I think I now have some authentic love for my parents. It is like I have done a full circle. I started at a challenging point of questioning my love for them and blaming them for my anorexia and depression. I began to question their infallibility, which caused my image of them to be shattered. Hatred and anger towards my parents emerged which eventually gave way to feeling numb.

Following this was a desire to have them out of my life completely. In this way I could manage them, even have some good feelings towards them from having resolved the past. To let them live on in my life was, and sometimes still is, frightening. Although I know they love me, they continue to give inconsistent messages that do not match what I am being told in therapy – which is the root of my problem is my parents. Now, at least sometimes, I feel love towards them. How is this possible? Aren't they the ogres in my story?

My eating is increasingly less of an issue. When I think about it I am surprised at how normal my response to food has become. I am now usually eating with genuine hunger, and treat foods are being eaten in normal ways and amounts.

Wednesday 23 August 1995

Yesterday I had my purse stolen from Ruby's stroller while she and I were in town. Once home, I sat on the floor in a corner sobbing. I was angry with myself for letting this happen and berated myself for being incompetent and untrustworthy. I did not think I should even exist. How had I dared to previously think I had a right to live?

Because I lost thirteen dollars cash, I now feel the need to make up for it. To deny myself milk, deny myself warmth of the heater and electric blanket. Although I am not physically debilitated today, my feelings and beliefs remain unchanged. Fortunately, I have an appointment to see Carmia today.

Carmia asked me if the need I now have to compensate for the loss of thirteen dollars, comes from the decision I made as a child to satisfy others, compensate and take responsibility? This still seems to make it my parents fault. Maybe it's mine. If I over-react to losing a few dollars - how would I fare losing family? Fear flows so fast when I consider losing Ruby, or Jack.

*****

In September of 1995, when I had been making great strides on writing a book, I discovered I was once again pregnant! I was overjoyed. It was such a thrilling prospect to be having another baby birthed around the same time that my book, hopefully, would be published. This pregnancy however, was not to last, and at fifteen weeks gestation I miscarried. Losing the baby was devastating. I kept thinking… its not suppose to happen like this!

We decided to name this child Jade. I bought a special plant and pot, and buried Jade under this special plant. I called the plant my 'Jade plant.'

The emotions of grief and loss were heavy, but my 'Jade plant,' that was an inside plant, brought me great comfort each time I looked at it. And, just as I had commenced journalling for Ruby from the time I knew I was pregnant with her, I began journalling for Jade. In Jade's journal I shared my heart and wrote all I thought and felt, and all I wanted Jade to know. I wrote until I had nothing left to write and the ache in my heart had eased. My 'Jade plant' and Jade's journal were special and healing touchstones for me.

The added emotion for me with the loss of Jade, was a fear that my book might abort too. I had not realized how the writing of a book was like going through something of a gestation also, with a birthing process of publication at the end.

Birthing Pains

Another even more spectacular surprise then came….

Only two months after losing Jade, **I was again pregnant!** I certainly had anxiety about whether this child would also miscarry, but I put my trust in Yehovah as well as I could. Once I got passed the first three months of pregnancy, I relaxed and had more peace and confidence that our second little girl would be born.

And so just a few weeks after the book was published in 1996, Ruby became a big sister to Charlotte. Book and baby both birthed - alive and well! Two years later, our son Levi was born.

*****

I did not know what response would come with the book's publication. After the gestation months of writing, the birthing process had happened with a book launch and The Salvation Army putting out a press release. This was to immediately springboard me into the various calls from radio stations in New Zealand and Australia for radio interviews. There were papers around New Zealand that printed reviews. The Capital's paper met with me to do a full-page feature article and photo, as did New Zealand's famous *NZ Woman's Weekly* magazine.

*****

CHAPTER 8

In The Pit

For my soul is full of troubles,
And my life draws near to the grave.
I am counted with those who go down to the pit;
I am like a man who has no strength.
Psalm 88:3-4

Only in Psychiatry is [brain] damage and dysfunction used as treatment! *(p.16) Despite more than 200 years of intensive research, no commonly diagnosed psychiatric disorders have been proven to be either genetic or biological in origin... (p.17)*

There are no known abnormalities in the brains of people who routinely seek help from psychiatrists... (p.xxiii)

Peter Breggin - Brain Disabling Treatments in Psychiatry

In 1998, I had once again spiraled into depression. Jack decided, in consultation with my doctors, that Electro-Convulsive Therapy (Electro-Shock Treatment) was just what I needed to snap me out of my depression. I had been re-diagnosed to have *Treatment Resistant Depression*, which was necessary in order to use Electroshock.

I'd had suicidal depression and anorexia, and I had recovered from both. For the past five years I had been in therapy, and it had served me well. I had my ups and downs of course, but I had made progress with overcoming depression, anxiety and anorexia. I had three children who I mothered and cared for. They were a daily joy to me. I picked up my work as a Salvation Army minister. I wrote a book and had it published to great acclaim. It was in demand enough to require a second printing. I received hundreds of letters from those who had been personally helped by my book, or seeking help for family and friends. I had established and led an eating disorder support group. I had led a young woman's accountability group. I also did a series of talks in my daughter's school, alleviating a problem of bullying in class. I was not *treatment resistant*!

At this point, the anorexia that had helped me cope with the depression, had been resolved. Or at least, had gone into 'remission.' [The Anorexia however, would later re-emerge to once again help me cope with the depression.]

Although I had taken a long and critical look at the Church and the usefulness of their approach to mental health issues, I had not lost my faith. During the times of deep despair, depression and disease, I never questioned Yeshua's reality or power. What I doubted was whether He would penetrate the prison I was in. I felt like I was in a bubble He could not enter. Had I gone beyond the point of no return? Was I past Yeshua's help? Nonetheless, it was my enduring faith in Yehovah-Yeshua that got me through the hospitalizations, suicidal episodes and the hopelessness of anorexia. When I was not strong enough to hold on to Him, He held on to me! This left me with a positive message for those suffering through similar circumstances.

Jack and I would both preach in our Salvation Army Corps (church), and my testimony and recovery reached many in the congregation. As well as this, I was invited to speak at various conferences in New Zealand and Australia. There were newspaper stories, radio and TV interviews. Maybe Jack struggled with his own sense of relevance. Jack had said to me that when I preached, people would respond to me emotionally, but when he preached no one, it seemed, responded. I emotionally connected with people. I had many good friends. People were drawn to me. It was not the same for Jack.

I was experiencing Jack's intermittent reinforcement, where he would give me intense affection and approval, and then alternate it with his disapproval, power, control and abuse. So while Jack and I had a deep emotional attachment, it was not based on love as I had thought. I equated the relationship to love, but it lacked mutual care and respect. My emotions were manipulated by Jack whose goal it was to exploit, not to reciprocate genuine love. The relationship was based on toxic influence, not love.

Eventually, this once again brought me into another phase of acute depression. This was a recurring pattern. I had attempted suicide two times and been hospitalized twice. Each time I fought my way back to health. Then Jack's manipulative behavior to exploit - rather than reciprocate genuine love - would eventually send me into another tailspin.

So it was at this point, Jack signed the consent to give me ECT…

*****

2024 Looking Back:
It is strange to think that this time, it would be deemed *'necessary'* to give me ECT!

My consent for ECT was neither sought nor given. But Jack agreed to ECT - so I submitted to it. I was never asked. Jack made the decision, not me. It was indicative of the mental hold Jack had on me, to assume the decision-making power over such a critically important treatment decision. I could have made my own decisions but did not. A critical part of me was still giving all my power over to Jack. That was the real problem underlying my mental illness.

The reason I was re-diagnosed with *Treatment Resistant Depression* is that ECT is not prescribed for depression - unless all other options have failed. Nor is ECT prescribed for anorexia, anxiety, domestic abuse, broken bones, or pneumonia. All of these issues have a cause. Running high voltage electricity through the brain does not affect the cause of any of these issues. Would a doctor agree to ECT for his alcohol problem, for example? One should hope not. Alcoholism is not cured by electric current through the brain. ECT is recommended when the psychiatric establishment has no answers.

Electro-Shock does not heal broken bones or pneumonia. These issues have a cause. Electro-Shock does not heal emotional or sexual abuse. These have a cause. Electro-Shock does not heal depression. It has a cause. Electro-Shock does not heal anorexia. Anorexia has a cause.

Electro-Shock causes brain injury. The psychiatric claim is that Electro-Shock changes "chemical imbalances" in the patient's brain - producing behavioral changes that are positive. Those "chemical imbalances" are never specified so they can never be verified. What Electro-Shock does, is to injure the brain, making the patient more docile - a result that is pleasing and helpful - except to the patient. Patients no longer complain. Problem solved.

Many doctors argue there is no such thing as *Treatment Resistant Depression*. In many cases, the patient has been massively drugged and switched from drug to drug. The reality is that they have been Drug Damaged as well - which can be as damaging as Electro-Shock. In my case, I had been on many medications and combinations of medications for depression for years. Doctors, as well as therapists, had also ignored the cause of my depression - domestic abuse - which had previously brought about my anorexia.

*****

ECT is a hugely controversial intervention. I prefer to call it Electro-Shock, as ECT implies that it is a healing medical therapy, which it is not. Using an acronym such as ECT denies its reality by cloaking it, so that it is unrecognized. It may even sound benign, just another healing treatment. Administering Electro-Shock causes trauma and dysfunction to the brain.

Jack consented to me having fifteen rounds of Electro-Shock over a period of seven and a half weeks while an inpatient of the Wellington Psychiatric Unit. I was not adequately informed about the risks. I did not have in my possession at any time, written information about this controversial experimental barbaric 'procedure' that was being inflicted on me. In any case, ECT is routinely described as "safe and effective." Emotional and sexual abuse is not treated by ECT.

Emotional and sexual abuse have a known cause. Running voltage through the brain in no way changes that cause. That is why the euphemism *Treatment Resistant Depression* was used to justify it.

Brain Injury is not a treatment.
It is inhumane. It is not medicine!

The truth is, there is no informed consent. Electro-Shock "treatment" is brain damage. In what world is brain injury a treatment? Textbooks describe ECT as changing the architectural structure of the brain, clearing away tissue, and causing cell death. Therefore informed consent would require being told that ECT is "cell death" - brain damage - but no one tells a patient that. Informed consent would require being told that ECT will result in cognitive dysfunction and memory loss, but patients are not told this.

Permanent memory loss and permanent damage to cognitive functioning are real physical effects which are life altering in a 'shocking' way. I had a right to know these things, especially since this treatment was dangerous and permanent brain damage is the result. One of the arguments given is that the patient is sedated so they do not feel the Electro-Shock. Patients are strapped down and given muscle relaxant - but there are still violent convulsions. It raises the question, if someone damages your brain and you never feel a thing - is your brain still damaged?

Patients do not get better as a result of ECT. They become more docile because they are brain damaged. Obviously, compliance is considered an improvement for difficult patients.

Tragically, ECT has been dramatically overused as a cure-all for many mental and behavioral disorders. Originally it was used for misbehaving children or promiscuous teenage girls. **Far from going out of style, ECT is now used more than ever before!** There are continued calls to extend the use of ECT to yet other disorders. Despite the profound ignorance surrounding ECT and its usefulness, or lack of it, it is still considered by many to be a cure-all. It is being steadily applied to more and more disorders that the psychiatric establishment does not know how to deal with.

Electro-Shock was a life-changing, shattering experience. I paid a vicious price. For example, I lost many memories of events in my relationship with my children. The outcome of the Electro-Shock to my brain was devastating - both in the short and long term. It left me brain damaged - referred to as Acquired Brain Injury (ABI) or Traumatic Brain Injury (TBI). After many years, I still live with effects of brain injury.

After a surgical procedure, one is stitched up, given antibiotics, and checked on around the clock. If there are adverse reactions, re-injury, torn stitches, or other complications - they are dealt with. However, after ECT, there is no aftercare, only a series of more rounds of brain injury.

When someone sustains a head injury, due to a sports or motor vehicle accident for instance, and this causes a concussion and bleeding, there is the initial emergency care. Ongoing treatment and rehabilitative care is also given for the traumatic brain injured patient.

In psychiatry however, if a patient has brain injury (from ECT), it is prescribed that the patient continues to have their head violently concussed twice a week for six weeks. I, and others who have received ECT were not given rehabilitative care, or counseling for the injury - only multiple continuing sessions of re-injury, before being left on our own to sink or swim with the effects of brain damage.

How can the psychiatric establishment give rehabilitative brain injury care and therapeutic counseling for ECT, when they have sworn it was "safe and effective?" Legally, that would be clear proof of the lies and mis-statements used to convince or coerce patients, and or their families, into using the brain-damaging ECT "*Treatment.*" Doctors would be legally responsible for the damage to the patient's brain. It would end the practice.

This also explains the lack of pre- and post- testing of memory and mental abilities before and after ECT. I was on my own in this damaged condition in an already abusive marriage. Spouses often divorce an ECT recipient, and ECT often destroys a patient's professional abilities to the point they can no longer pursue their career. I was not able to work as a Registered Nurse (R.N.) ever again!

Medical doctors take an oath of ethics called the Hippocratic Oath, ***"First, do no harm!"***

What happened to that Hippocratic oath?

Aftershock

Prior to Electro-Shock, I had been an R.N., a Salvation Army officer (minister), and a mother. At the time, my youngest child Levi was a baby, and since I was breastfeeding him, my psychiatrist admitted us both to the Wellington Psychiatric Unit. Levi was in a room with his own special nurse around the clock, and my room was next to Levi's. The decision was made for me to stop breastfeeding Levi and have his nurse bottle feed him. Then the hospital psychiatrist advised Jack that ECT was what I needed. I needed extensive help to care for my young children. I was unable to write or present publicly. Eventually I had to resign as a Salvation Army minister. I was not able to work as an R.N. again - even though I tried. Ultimately, and most significantly, I lost my marriage and children.

Physiological outcomes for me: If you attend fifteen social events over an eight-week period, you have fifteen sets of memories. Right? I had fifteen excursions to the pink room for Electro-Shock and have little to no memory of these times. I will tell you what I do remember. I do remember being taken from the ward in a wheelchair to a pink room. I do remember lying on an operating table. I do remember being asked to count backwards as I succumbed to the general anesthetic.

I do remember that I was quiet, obliging, depressed. I was not scared. I do remember tears rolling down my face, tears of shame. I do remember being willing for them to do whatever they wanted. I did not much care, as long as I did not have to do anything, think anything or feel anything emotionally. I do remember sitting in the wheelchair back in my room on the ward, being offered a light snack.

Though I do not remember eating it. I do remember feeling very tired, as if I had been through a major battle.

I do ***not*** remember being given the muscle relaxant, or being strapped down, or having the electrodes placed on my head. I do ***not*** remember having something put in my mouth to stop me biting my tongue, or seeing the volt meter switched on, or seeing the volt meter dial move in a sweeping arch from the far left to the right. I do ***not*** remember my body convulsing as the electric current surged through my brain.

I know these things happened because some years later when I was attempting to return to nursing, I was on a clinical placement at a different hospital and was tasked with accompanying a young woman to a similar pink room and watched as she underwent Electro-Shock. This was a hugely conflicting experience for me. There were violent convulsions! It did require a tongue protector, so the patient did not bite her tongue. The patient was strapped down to kept her from interfering with the Electro-Shock. That was me on the table!

Being back in the psychiatric ward subsequent to my Electro-Shock 'treatments,' I became easily disorientated in many surroundings. I was told I needed help to know how to get to the bathroom and then to my room. I needed help to know how to get to the Occupational Therapy room, which I had known very well from previous admissions and outpatient care.

I have limited recall of other events too, throughout those eight weeks I was in the psychiatric unit. The memories of this time are patchy and incomplete. I knew some things because they were later told to me. One was of Levi in his Jolly Jumper in the doorway of his room, and me sitting on the floor watching him bounce. I remember something of what his room looked like, and his tall steel hospital baby cot. I think it is from my own recall that I had a bath with Charlotte who was a toddler. Jack had brought her to visit because she was missing me and upset. The staff allowed her to share some close time with me - to calm us both down.

I was molested on the ward by another patient, during the weeks of the Electro-Shock sessions. I had to be rescued by the staff. I only know about it because the staff were required by law to notify Jack. What actually happened? What kind of molestation was it? I do not know, but I had to be rescued. I asked what happened, and was told, *"best you don't know - good thing you have no memory of it."* Clearly, it was a very serious event, but I have no memory of it.

I have a fuzzy memory of Jack having sex with me in the visitor's restroom just outside the ward. I have another memory of Jack taking me under a tree on the hospital grounds. On both occasions, Jack was visiting me and requested permission to take me out of the ward for a walk while it was night and dark outside. The staff allowed me to leave the ward because they assumed Jack would care for me.

In my right mind I would never have permitted sex in a public area. It happened because of the brain damage caused by the Electro-Shock. Jack clearly considered docility to be a beneficial effect of the treatment. Strangely, I was not considered capable of giving consent to ECT - yet my consent to risqué sex on the grounds was assumed. I felt like my only value to Jack was as a sex object. He did not care about the damage to my brain.

Abuse is fueled by entitlement

Husbands who sexually abuse their wives do it because they love themselves and their own pleasure to such an extent that they have no self-control (Consider 2 Timothy 3:2–5). They are willing to be reckless and heartless.
Patrick Weaver - The Exodus Project

Once home, I saw a beautiful mosaic papier-mâché pot in my daughter Ruby's bedroom. I asked her where it had come from. She looked at me strangely and said that we (she and I) had made it together at the hospital (Occupational Therapy).

Following Electro-Shock I tired easily and had a great need to sleep a lot. I was tired so much of the time. I had difficulty comprehending information and instructions. My speech was slow and halting. I struggled to get my words and thoughts out. I had extreme noise sensitivity, even being among regular 'life-noise' was like being in the middle of a war zone. In these danger zones, like a restaurant or church, I was not able to converse or even think. Music venues or movie theaters were impossible for me. It was an overwhelming assault on my senses, even my person. When I had tried to endure these experiences, I quickly became exhausted and distressed by the experience, and desperate to leave.

ECT resulted in severe memory loss and diminished cognitive functioning. I lost complete memories in the early days. There was one occasion a young woman came up to me at church and conversed with me as if I knew her. I cautiously asked if I knew her from somewhere. I was embarrassed to find out that I actually knew her very well. She was a friend and had been in our home many times.

Some memories were only fragments. Our memories are what make up a significant part of who we are. No one has the right to deny another of the right to their life and experience.

I lost a great deal of desire, enjoyment and capacity for creativity. Reading and learning new things had now become an insurmountable challenge. I struggled to comprehend or find information. I could not concentrate or hold necessary information to grasp anything complex. My ability to absorb or retain new information decreased to almost non-existent. I could not follow the news on television or keep up with a conversation. I lost my ability to follow rapid speech and follow instructions. I became very good at giving the impression of understanding and following conversations with nods and and a few carefully placed words, questions or comments. I could not commit things to memory. I constantly needed to re-learn and re-know things. I would get hopelessly lost in a small and previously known area, and I could watch a movie many times over and swear it was the first time I had ever seen it! I was actually like the character in the movie *'50 First Dates'* who could never remember what happened the day before! All these things created a great deal of stress and anxiety for me, and consternation for others.

As one might expect, my sense of self-worth was affected, instigating something of an identity crisis. Who was I now? What was I even capable of? No one, including Jack, seemed to understand how much damage the Electro-Shock had done to my brain and how much more difficult it was for me to function normally. I had not gained relief from my depression as a result of Electro-Shock. Instead, it left me with a deeper depression and suicidality that I had to get over.

2024 Looking Back:
Post ECT, patients who commit suicide usually do so the first week after treatment. If a patient does not have the ability to cope with life before ECT, they certainly have much less ability after ECT. What they do have, as a result of ECT - was the same thing I had - exacerbated hopelessness. I attempted suicide twice more after my Electro-Shocks. Over many years I had wondered if I would ever be capable of regular life again. Life was way too overwhelming, too demanding and too complex. I felt incompatible with life.

Things I have learned about ECT as a Nurse and Professional Mental Health Advocate

"There are no known abnormalities in the brains of people who routinely seek help from psychiatrists and who become diagnosed with disorders like ADHD, schizophrenia, and major depressive disorder." (Breggin, 2008 p.xxiii)

"Electroshock treatment causes permanent brain damage and dysfunction." (p.xxv)

"Antidepressant drugs cause a spectrum of stimulant or activation effects - including agitation, hostility, aggression, and mania as well as crashing into depression and suicidality…" (p.xxvii)

"The last two decades have seen escalating reliance on psychiatric drugs…" (p.xxix)

"This drug revolution views psychiatric medications as far more helpful than harmful… they are said to correct chemical imbalances in the brain." (p.xxix)

"Drug companies heavily promote that unproven speculation that the problems they treat are biological in origin and result from biochemical imbalances." (p.xxx)

"Most health care providers… have been taught to believe that psychiatric disorders have known biological and genetic causes. Despite more than 200 years of intensive research, no commonly diagnosed psychiatric disorders have been proven to be either genetic or biological in origin, including the diagnostic categories of schizophrenia, major depressive disorder and bipolar disorder, the various anxiety disorders, and childhood disorders such as attention-deficit hyperactivity. At present, there are no known bio-chemical imbalances in the brain of typical psychiatric patients - until they are given psychiatric drugs." (p.17)

"The failure to demonstrate the existence of any brain abnormality in psychiatric patients, despite decades of intensive effort, suggests that these defects do not exist." (p.17)

"Instead of correcting biochemical imbalances, psychiatric drugs cause them, sometimes permanently." (Breggin, 2008, p.1)

"The brain-disabling concept as a whole states that all psychiatric treatments - drugs, Electroshock, and lobotomy - work by disrupting the function of the brain and mind, creating effects that are then interpreted (or mis-interpreted) as improvements." (p.1)

Four Basic Brain-Disabling Principles. (Breggin, 2008, pp.2-4)

I. All bio-psychiatric treatments share a common mode of action; the disruption of normal brain function.

II. All bio-psychiatric interventions cause generalized brain dysfunction.

III. Bio-psychiatric treatments exert their therapeutic effect by impairing higher human functions, including emotional responsiveness, social sensitivity, self-awareness or self-insight, autonomy, and self-determination. More drastic effects include apathy, euphoria and mania, and lobotomy-like indifference.

IV. Each bio-psychiatric treatment produces its essential or brain-disabling effect on all people, including normal volunteers and patients with varied psychiatric diagnoses.

"A lobotomy… suppresses the limbic system and frontal lobe function, causing apathy and indifference. The patients no longer care enough to express their… symptoms, but they also no longer care about anything. It is a global deactivation… This is a pillar of the brain-disabling concept: that psychiatric drugs work by disabling the higher centers of the brain!" (p.5)

"Patients respond to brain-disabling treatments with their own psychological reactions such as apathy, euphoria, compliance, or resentment." (p.7)

"To the extent that a physical disorder of the brain affects the individual, currently available bio-psychiatric interventions will worsen or add to the disorder." (p.7)

"Electroshock and lobotomy are justified on the grounds that they correct biochemical imbalances… In reality, **all currently available bio-psychiatric interventions cause direct harm to the brain** and hence to the mind, without correcting any known malfunction." (p.8)

"The pharmaceutical industry has lobbied hard to convince the U.S. Congress, the health profession, and the public that emotional problems such as depression and anxiety are biological in origin." (p.8) [Note: *chemical imbalances* would be an example of biological origin.]

"Individual bio-psychiatric treatments are not specific for particular mental disorders." (p.8)

[Note: The *chemicals* which are supposedly *imbalanced* in the brain are never specified nor is any treatment offered to specifically treat that *imbalance*.]

"Physicians typically attribute their patients' worsening condition to 'mental illness' when in reality the patient is suffering from adverse drug reactions!" (p.9)

"*Anosognosia* refers to the capacity of brain damage to cause denial of lost function... a hallmark of central nervous disability from any cause." (p.11) [Note: For example, many drugs used include pain killers or sedatives producing euphoria. Few patients will complain of lost function while euphoric. It could be called the *Heroin Effect;* how many addicts refuse to acknowledge their worsening physical and mental state even when obvious to others?

It is called '*Medication Spellbinding*' (see *Medication Madness,* Breggin, 2009). "Spellbound individuals often feel as if they are doing better than ever when in reality they are doing worse."

[Note: It is critically important to be aware that the result of complaining about the effects of Electro-Shock treatment is to be given more Electro-Shock - an obvious factor in the numbers of patients who claim improvement after Electro-Shock!]

"Lobotomized or Electro-Shocked patients... have greatly impaired self-awareness... they are likely to report that they are doing better than they are." (p.12)

"The vast majority of problems routinely treated as so-called mental disorders do not remotely resemble diseases of the brain or body... to claim that an irrational or emotionally distressed state, however extreme, in itself amounts to impaired brain function is simply false." (p.18)

[Note: 'Impaired brain function' due to biological factors such as 'chemical imbalances' are the rationales used in giving psychiatric drugs, Electro-Shock, and surgical lobotomies.]

"The concepts of mental illness and mental disorder are misleading… none of the problems commonly treated by psychiatrists are genetic or biological in origin." (p.19)

"ECT is frequently used and retains enormous support within the medical profession." (p.217)

"Although studies have demonstrated that electro-convulsive therapy (ECT) is an effective and safe treatment for severe major depression, inaccurate perceptions of ECT contribute to lingering stigma and fear regarding its use." *Journal of the American Medication Association* (JAMA) September 12, 2007 - titled "Interest Surging in Electro-convulsive… therapy."

"This positive and even promotional attitude flies in the face of decades of research and heart-rending patient testimonials. The publication of this puff piece at this time is probably intended to counter yet one more recently published scientific study that demonstrated… electro-convulsive therapy (ECT) causes permanent brain dysfunction and damage, including widespread memory and cognitive deficits… **ECT greatly elevates the suicide risk, especially in the first week following treatment**… And finally, for the first time in history, an ECT malpractice case has been won in court!" (p.218)

Things I have experienced as a recipient of Electro-Shock Treatment

I was no longer the same person after Electro-Shock. It changed me - not just in the immediate time but for decades to come. **ECT is the rape of the soul!** This is not an overstatement. There were so many deficits I had that I was unaware of. ECT left me feeling diminished, shamed and anxious. I was already a disabled person - but now facing additional daily challenges.

My family had been told there were no long-term effects of ECT so they did not think to offer help or even discuss the support I might need because of the brain injury.

Later, a professional medical analysis concluded I had the brain damage comparable to someone in a high-speed car accident. This testing outcome was validating, yet for me there was no accident financial help. I was left having to support myself with no help whatsoever. It was overwhelming to the point of despair. Only my faith got me through the ordeal.

For years to come, I carried Electro-Shock as my shame. I did not speak of it to others for twenty-two years but simply explained my mental challenges to others as being a result of a brain injury. When they would ask how that happened, I would say I would prefer not to talk about it. I should have been honest, or even angry, but not ashamed at what was done to me. I had trusted in the medical profession to help me, but quite the opposite occurred. ECT is a horrific procedure, worthy of Dr. Mengele. Doctors vastly downplay any side effects. This is a deception. **Brain damage is not a side effect - it is the direct effect of ECT!** It is a criminal assault, and doctors should be held criminally liable for unethical practice and denying the risks. Above all, I realized that Jack had betrayed me!

When I tried to return to work as an R.N., I could not perform adequately under stress and lasting memory deficits. Electro-Shock erased a great deal of my learning, leaving me stressed and anxious. I was no longer patient-safe in my work. In time I did have a job as a nurse assistant in Australia. I was financially destitute having lost my nursing career. Instead of making more and more money with experience and seniority as a nurse, I was reduced to a fraction of the salary as a nurse assistant working part-time. I was chronically fatigued as a result of the Electro-Shock. I did not have the stamina for full-time work. I had years of simply struggling to survive.

ECT is touted as '*safe and effective,*' and any side effects will be short term. Not so. Electro-Shock is not safe. Furthermore, psychiatrists tout this as lifesaving, like the cardiac defibrillator. Yet in the case of the defibrillator there has been responsible testing of both the procedure and device. **Electro-Shock treatment has never had any FDA testing for safety or effectiveness!** Withholding this information from patients is inexcusable. As a result, many hospitals routinely use ECT leading to permanent disabilities.

As for ECT being '*effective*'... ECT makes patients more docile and therefore easier to control. This certainly did not help my domestic situation. Sexual docility exacerbated the control of Jack over me. It is not hard to imagine this contributed to his decision to seek it.

When I was breaking free from domestic abuse, my husband used my mental health disability and ECT history to take my children from me. I was traumatized, alone, alienated from most of my family because of my ex-husband, brain-injured, financially destitute, responsible for child-care payments, yet being kept from any contact with my children. It was devastating and demoralizing.

Electro-Shock was a life-changing experience for me. Even after twenty-six years, there are still disabilities to contend with. I have worked very hard to retrain my brain, learning alternative ways to remember things, and alternative ways to do things that would get me through. Repetition, routines, lists, notes, word associations... I believe this has created many new pathways in my brain.

I still have sensory, emotional and information overload challenges. My reading comprehension is difficult. I try to simplify life and avoid things that are too complex, chaotic or unpredictable. I need agreed limits or assurance that things are not going to get too big and overwhelming. I realize that at times, these needs might be perceived by others as me being rigid, or even boring, but the alternative is for me getting too close to the emotional edge. This is not a happy place for me. If I get pushed over the edge - it is disastrous!

I no longer trust medical and psychiatric doctors or the greater medical establishment. It is difficult for me to consent to any hospital care. I know there are many more people today who feel this way, as the medical and drug industries have further revealed themselves.

Before Electroshock I was a successful author. After Electro-Shock, it took me more than two decades to recover to the point I could attempt writing again. So do I believe that my experience of Electroshock can and is being redeemed in my life, just as every other event, experience, or outcome? Absolutely, but the cost and losses of recovery have been enormous!

2024 Spiritual Awakening:
In fact, during the process of writing this book and praying for inner healing for this distressing experience of ECT - my friend Lisa Townley was shown something by Yehovah. In her spirit, she saw me on the operation table while ECT was being administered. Yeshua was there with his body bent over to cover mine - shielding me from more permanent harm being inflicted by ECT - his body was draped over me like a prayer shawl! To know that Yeshua was with me in this way, was a precious and healing revelation for me.

The power of Yehovah to heal, is equal to none. NOTHING is impossible to Him! The greater the problem, the greater is His glory that is demonstrated!

When I consider Your Heavens, the work of Your fingers,
The moon and the stars, which You have ordained,

What is mankind that You are mindful of him,
And the son of man that You visit him?

For You have made him a little lower than Elohim [God],
And You have crowned him with glory and honor.

You have made him to have dominion over
the works of Your hands;
You have put all things under his feet...

Psalm 8:3-6

The Heavens and the Earth declare the glory of Yehovah and every creature within them are evidence of Yehovah's creative power and generosity of His love. But of all Yehovah's creations, perhaps the most amazing one is man's brain. It is an amazing feat of divine engineering. There are more connections among the brain's neurons than there are known stars in the universe!

The psalmist wonders, with recognizable emotion, why our Creator has made mankind, a little lower than Himself, and crowned us with glory and honor, and given us dominion over the works of His hands;

and has put all things [including Satan!] under our feet. With the brain that Yehovah has given us, we are capable of fulfilling the callings He has entrusted to us, and of fighting the good fight of faith. Hallelujah and amen!

*****

Healing Prayer by Lisa Townley:

(Use this prayer for anyone who has had ECT)

Yehovah, we come boldly before your throne.

Yeshua we come to You. You are our burden bearer.

Holy Spirit, You are our Comforter, in our time of grief.

We receive Your comfort for Cate. We know that one day the truth will be expressed to her children. Whether they come to it by reading this book, or if it is when they come to stand before You, the truth will be revealed to them. We ask that it would be done while on this Earth, so that there will be reconciliation.

We place the Blood of Yeshua on this book and over these circumstances. Yeshua we ask you to take the heaviness of this grief, that Cate feels. We release it to you. We ask you to heal the wounds that this grief has caused, and we receive your healing now.

Yehovah, You know all things. Nothing is hidden from You. All things are as day in Your presence. You know every clinic and institution that administers ECT. You know the wickedness behind it and the destruction it causes. I know that this breaks Your heart.

We thank you Yeshua that you are the Redeemer, Healer, and Deliverer. We thank you that you understand the torture and torment that every ECT patient has experienced. You fellowship with the suffering of those people. Yeshua, may every patient who has, or is experiencing ECT, know that you are near. May they turn to the Light of who you are. And as you have healed Cate, and brought about miraculous recovery in her brain and in her soul, we ask that you would bring that recovery and healing to every patient who has, or is, or who will experience ECT.

We ask You great Yehovah, our Healer, touch these beautiful people. Expose the wickedness of ECT and destroy its works and effects.

We ask You to forgive the medical system and industry, for inflicting physical and psychological abuse with the administration of ECT. For the raping of souls. As Yeshua prayed on the cross, "Father forgive them, for they don't know what they are doing."

We pray that you would remove the blinders. You would expose this, as you are exposing and expelling so many other wicked things right now in the world. We declare and decree that ECT will be exposed for what it is, and removed. It will be destroyed and stopped!

Yehovah, we need Your love, Your healing. Pour truth into this world. For all of the other experiences Cate has been through, we decree and declare that it shall be for Your glory, and that there MUST be redemption. We receive redemption of Cate's family - her children, grandchildren, great-grandchildren and great-great-grandchildren. We receive healing, deliverance, freedom, reconciliation and deliverance into her family. Truth **shall** *prevail in the mighty name of Yeshua.*

Yeshua, you taught us that when we pray, we are to pray with faith without any doubting - believing that we have received, and we shall move any mountains. So with our faith right now, we decree and declare reconciliation with ALL her family - her children, her grandchildren, her siblings, her nieces and nephews, and we decree and declare that it shall be, and we call it forth quickly.

Thank you Yeshua that nothing, absolutely nothing is impossible for us when we believe. So we ask you to keep on increasing our faith, that we shall stand and we shall see how great is Yehovah fighting this battle for us. We are only to stand still and believe.

Thank you Yehovah, thank you Yeshua, thank you Holy Spirit, thank you mighty angels, that you fight for us.

Cate: *And I decree and declare that I shall see Yehovah's goodness in the land of the living!* (Psalm 27:13)

CHAPTER 9

Stars in the Heavens

Remember Abraham, Isaac, and Jacob, Your servants,
to whom You swore by Your own self, and said to them,
'I will multiply your descendants as the stars of Heaven;
and all this land that I have spoken of I give to your descendants,
and they shall inherit it forever.'
Exodus 32:13

Ruby was born in 1993, one week after her due date. She was born healthy, well and absolutely beautiful! I had managed to keep good health throughout the pregnanc, and this was well rewarded with a beautiful baby girl in my arms! I continued with therapy throughout this time and beyond, and I loved being a mother. It was what I had always wanted and dreamed of, and becoming a mother gave me tremendous joy!

Ruby was every bit as determined as she was bright and beautiful. Determined not to sleep. Determined not to be put down in her cot. Determined to always be moving. Simply determined to be determined. At fifteen weeks old she was standing unaided. At nine months old she was walking as competently as any adult.

Charlotte was born in 1996, and her entry into the world was an undiagnosed footling breech birth. This surprise made for some touch-and-go moments in the delivery suite, but she and I made it through—albeit with me later needing some surgical structural repairs. Charlotte was also healthy, well and absolutely beautiful.

Charlotte's easy temperament was a contrast to Ruby's. She was responsive to parenting - calm, cuddly, happy, adaptable and easy to soothe. Her delightful personality brought much joy to me and the family with her peaceable and gentle nature and was ever so cute with her curly blonde hair!

Levi was born in 1998, when Charlotte was almost two years old. He was born by Caesarean section and was born every bit as healthy and strong and gorgeous as his sisters. Levi's temperament was a combo - both easy and difficult to parent! He was charming, endearing, strong-willed, cuddly, adventurous, determined, fun-loving and fun.

Levi was a natural-born climber and my little 'Houdini'! When he was ten months old, he pulled a jail-break when he figured out how to climb right out of his crib. He was a repeat offender, and it was impossible to keep him in his crib. To keep him safe until we could come up with a better solution, we put his mattress on the floor, laid Levi on the mattress, and then put the upturned crib over the top of Levi. That did the trick! The solution we then came up with, was to use a sleep wrap for babies. This is a piece of fabric wrapped completely around the mattress with an additional piece of attached fabric securely wrapped around Levi's mid torso and fastened with Velcro. His arms, legs and hips were free to move naturally.

The wide piece of stuck together Velcro was meant to be much too difficult for a baby to pull apart and get themselves out of, but not for Levi, it turned out. Each time after putting him to bed he would rip the Velcro apart, and out of bed he would go! Neither was it too hard for him to get out of his bed when I additionally secured it with two safety pins, or, when I also further secured it with a double knotted dish towel over the double-safety-pinned Velcro. To my dismay and wonderment, he got them all undone!

Ruby, Charlotte and Levi were all full-term babies and were all fully breastfed. From even before they were born, I journaled about them. I continued these journals for them throughout all the years I had with them as their mother.

*****

Ruby, Charlotte and Levi were such a blessing to me with their different personalities, strengths, and giftings.

Right from the beginning, Ruby was a confident and independent kind of gal, who did not mind going against the flow, and this made for some challenging parenting! Throughout her childhood and teenage years, she loved to learn, express her mind and debate. She was an avid reader and a prolific artist—painting and drawing. She was very funny with her clever and quick wit and was academically accomplished. Ruby had a pragmatic way of thinking and was not easily dissuaded from anything she believed or set her mind on. She was highly motivated to achieve goals that she set for herself, or to achieve goals that came with financial reward.

Charlotte was kind, loving and tender-hearted to everyone, and as long as she was fed and had enough sleep, she was a happy camper. Charlotte had happy-humor and with her creative flare she could take anything that was regular or ordinary and transform it into something extraordinary. That is, she would *Charlotte-ise* her clothes, her hair, her bedroom walls, her door, her schoolbooks etc. Charlotte excelled at school and was a dream student for her teachers. Charlotte was thoughtful and reflective, loyal and committed. With her gentle spirit, she attracted many friends, and friends were important to her. She was most content when those around her were being happy, kind and loving to each other.

Levi was all about fun, action and adventure. He was always pushing his physical strengths and pushing the boundaries. He did not like missing out on anything and would get very frustrated and upset if things were not going his way or if his fun was reigned in. He was a charmer through and through, and could charm his way into anyone's heart - and out of trouble! - with his smile and endearing ways. Levi could annoy and play pranks on his big sisters, but they loved him. It was hard for anyone not to love Levi! He had a great mind, and even as a young child he was demonstrating his mechanical intelligence.

Levi would say *"yes"* to everything new to try or place to go, while Ruby was more likely to say *"no,"* and Charlotte would be considered and cautious. Charlotte and Levi were my cuddle-bugs, wanting and giving all manner of physical love and affection. Generally, Ruby did not want or need this. Ruby and Charlotte liked having alone time reading, while Levi always wanted company, and he would rather have me read a book to him!

Money motivated Ruby into action. Charlotte was motivated by everyone around her getting along and being loving towards each other. Levi would get tasks done as long as it could be made fun, or there was a promised reward of something fun, waiting at the end. Ruby learned to play the guitar, Charlotte learned to play the recorder and sang in a choir, Levi learned to play the trumpet. Sports-wise, Ruby and Charlotte played netball and Levi played rugby. They all did well in Friday night swimming training. They all rode scooters and bikes, and roller bladed.

As well as journaling for my children, I also gathered for them over their childhood all sorts of memorabilia of their lives, that were kept in their own big individual *special boxes*. In them were baby items, their school and sport awards and certificates, their birthday cards I had made for them, their special artwork and creations, mementos from special family holidays, their own photo albums I put together etc…

Since Ruby was a book-lover and prolific reader since pre-school age, she and I made many visits to the local library, reading and checking out books to bring home. Later I did this with Charlotte and Levi too. When Ruby became accomplished at chapter-book reading, it was not uncommon for her to take home two or even three dozen books from a library visit, that she would avidly devour over a week.

Ruby drew, painted and created just as prolifically and well. So much so, that I thought to have art exhibitions for her work - we had to share it around somehow! Charlotte and Levi's artwork too. I would title, prepare and catalogue the children's artwork, sometimes as many as a hundred masterpieces! Adult family and friends would be invited to the Exhibition Day. Our living room furniture got moved into other rooms of the house for these occasions, so that freestanding partitions could be placed for the artwork to be displayed on. I laminated many pieces of artwork. Some special pieces were for display only, or could be purchased as a print from the original. Many other pieces were simply sold. These were fun and rewarding occasions that were every bit worth the great effort made. The funds raised by the children's efforts, would be used to purchase more art supplies for their wonderful expressions of art to continue.

As Ruby was a very confident child, she had every expectation that people would want and value her artwork. Which they did. I think for Charlotte and Levi, these art exhibitions gave them both a greater knowing that the loving and caring adults in their lives believed in them and valued what they could do.

Charlotte loved stories and became an accomplished reader just like her big sister. I have some treasured memories of each and all of the children sitting on the big armchair with me engrossed in stories together. Charlotte was equally creative and had a wonderful imagination too. I would watch as she played with neighborhood children, or as she played dress-ups with her little brother Levi. As Charlotte got older, she loved to go thrift-store-shopping, as I did, to find unique and interesting clothes. She had a knack for customizing her clothes and wearing them with flare. I taught Charlotte to use the sewing machine and how to make some superb chocolate cakes and lasagna!

Levi excelled in hard skills, imagination and making plans! He loved to have me read to him or to tell him made-up stories. Lego, hammer and nails, nuts and bolts, arm wrestling, skateboarding, back rubs, and bribing his sisters was the stuff of 'fun' for him! Together, Levi and I liked making sushi, bike rides, and swimming out to a pontoon and jumping off it to see who could make the biggest splash. Besides teaching Levi how to ride a bike, I also taught him to knit and hand sew when he was only six or seven. He was very keen, very determined, and very good! He knit a scarf and he hand-sewed a patchwork baby quilt, with a bit of help from me, both of which he was very proud.

All three children earned pocket money for extra contributions to the household, and like I had done as a child, Charlotte and Levi put advertisement flyers in people's letter boxes. I helped and supported them with.

Family activities included rollerblading, biking and scootering together around Oriental Parade, watching family movies, and eating chocolate. We also managed to go on holiday to different parts of New Zealand, Australia and North America.

*****

Jade was my second pregnancy and the child I never got to hold, love, care for, or know, having miscarried this child fifteen weeks into the pregnancy. I did not get to have those same sweet memories of Jade. This was the strange thing though… Whenever I was out with my children and needed to round them up, or just check their whereabouts, I would do a mental count of them — 1,2,3… and then have a fleeting moment of concern, that there should be one more, or that I had lost one! While I only had the three— Ruby, Charlotte and Levi— I think I subconsciously was always looking for my other child. Jade was my fourth, my missing child.

*****

2024 Looking Back:
I was seen by others as a good, loving and creative mother. Jack would also tell me, and write in Mother's Day cards, that I was a good mother to our children. I know I am blessed to have so many sweet memories of them, yet for many years these memories have tormented me. The extreme alienation from my children that I was to experience became hugely conflicting with these memories and experiences.

The love and joy of motherhood contrasted to the experience of dark depression that would overtake me, as a result of the power and control being exerted over me by Jack in the marriage. I would keep myself well enough for extended lengths of time, and then I would crash into poor mental health.

The Power and Control Wheel

THE DULUTH MODEL POWER & CONTROL WHEEL
Produced & distributed by:
National Center on Domestic and Sexual Violence, USA.

Physical v Psychological Violence

"Physical and sexual assaults, or threats to commit them, are the most apparent forms of domestic violence and are usually the actions that allow others to become aware of the problem.

However, regular use of other abusive behaviors by the batterer, when reinforced by one or more acts of physical violence, make up a larger system of abuse. Although physical assaults may occur only once or occasionally, they instill threat of future violent attacks and allow the abuser to take control of the woman's life and circumstances.

The Duluth Model Power & Control diagram is a particularly helpful tool in understanding the overall pattern of abusive and violent behaviors, which are used by a batterer to establish and maintain control over his partner. Very often, one or more violent incidents are accompanied by an array or these other types of abuse. They are less easily identifies, yet firmly establish a pattern of intimidation and control in the relationship."

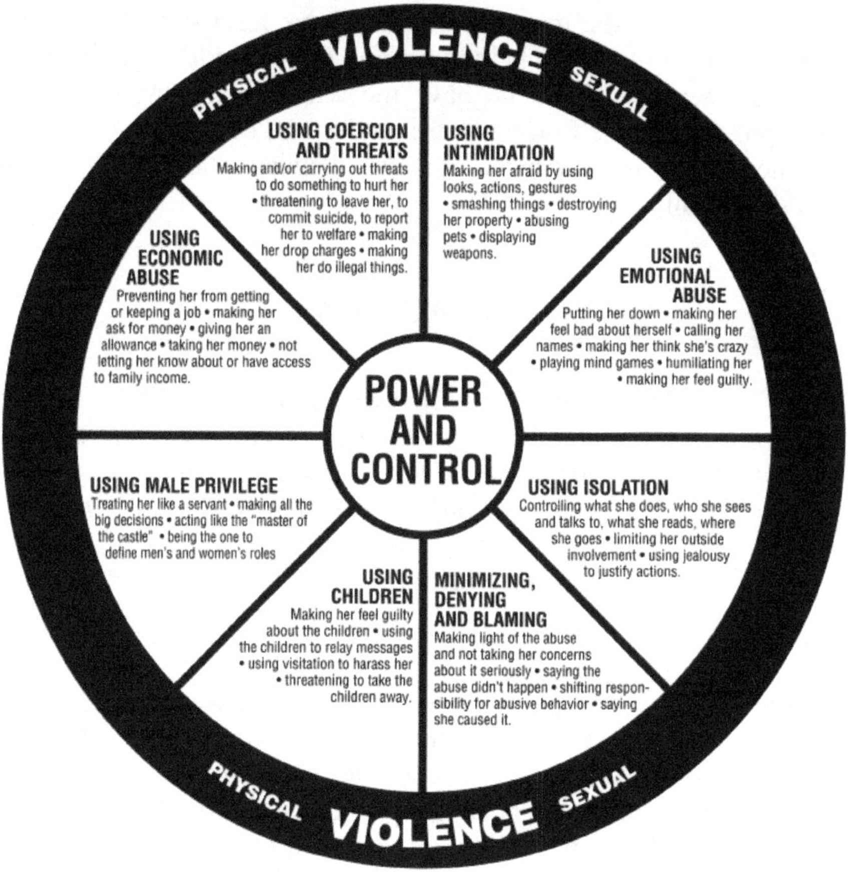

*****

Sexual abuse in marriage can result in severe outcomes for the victim - these include: Physical injury or harm, Emotional trauma and distress, Anxiety and depression, PTSD and other mental health issues, Difficulty forming healthy relationships in the future, Feeling shame, guilt, and self-blame.

There were times when Levi as a young child would climb into bed with Jack and I in the morning. I would have Levi snuggled up with me, and Jack would get in behind me and either digitally penetrate me or use his penis. Jack would have me with him in the shower. He would position himself on his knees under me, between my legs, and have me urinate over his head. This was disgusting and surreal to me. Yet it thrilled him.

Pornography

Her religious community not only encourage this
blanket forgiveness, but defines her forgiveness to mean she
must act as if he had never done any wrong. This level of
forgiveness they demand from her, body and soul, at all times.
It is her duty as a wife, and she takes it seriously.
Natalie Hoffman - Is It Me?

When all three of our children were school aged, our youngest Levi only just in school, we had a family personal computer (PC). This was before the time that either Jack or I had a laptop, and our children certainly did not have one back in those days! So, the family PC was used by Jack, and by me, and by our children for their homework and learning. One day when I was working on the PC, a pornographic website and pictures popped up on the screen. I was outraged and perturbed, and told Jack about it that evening. I was not thinking at all that it was any more than a random happening that we did not want reoccurring. After all, our children were using this PC. Jack agreed with me, and nothing more was said. Then a short while later when I was again using the PC, other pornographic images filled the screen. Suddenly I was suspicious. That night I told Jack this had happened again, and I wanted to know if he knew anything about why. I asked, was he watching pornography on the PC?

I remember catching a guilty look in his eyes. My naïveté was shattered! These were our children he was endangering. I was mortified! Suddenly the tables had turned. I was no longer the submissive and powerless girl-child to Jack. The mother bear was awakened. I was no longer unaware. Now I was addressing him about something where he had to give an account of himself to me! This was such a strange and unexpected predicament for us both. I had not ever experienced this dynamic before. Jack had always been the powerful one who was right and who decided things - and I was the submissive follower who did not know what was best. It was this imbalance of power, coercion and control that created the abuse in our marriage. I had given my power away to Jack - in that moment I took it back!

I was shocked to know the truth that he had been watching pornography, and that he had been using the family PC that our children also used! I told him in no uncertain terms that he had to get rid of anything that would bring these images up again. Jack said he would. He was caught out. It was an uncomfortable situation for him. I never mentioned this again to him. I trusted that he would do as he said he would. I trusted that was the end of pornography. I trusted…

*****

Like a wound that never heals because the source of the infection is never identified and dealt with, anorexia, depression and anxiety were to be conditions that would hound me throughout the course of my marriage to various degrees. I would continually cycle through illness into reasonable health, then back into illness followed by reasonable health again.

Publishing my book had been a springboard into a string of radio and television interviews in New Zealand and Australia, and speaking at a national counselor's conference. The ministry roles, sermon preparation or employment tasks I took on, happened in the evening hours or when our children were in bed, or when they were at school.

She will work hard at raising the family, taking care of the home, and prudently spending. She will also work hard at her career to bring in monetary value. No gift is too great in her mind. It is all a pleasure to give... This works wonderfully for the man who views her as his servant...
Natalie Hoffman - Is It Me?

The Salvation Army gave me the opportunity to establish an eating support program, where I would meet each week with a group of young women from the community who were struggling with Anorexia nervosa or Bulimia Nervosa. In this time I also accepted an invitation to lead a workshop at a national Youth Suicide Prevention conference, hosted by The Salvation Army. I also presented / facilitated two training days for the staff of a couple of Salvation Army addiction programs regarding eating disorders as they might sometimes present with addictions.

I undertook various roles as a Salvation Army Minister - preaching, facilitating a young women's accountability group, teaching emotional health classes at a girl's high school, as well as working in and offering pastoral care in one our Salvation Army Thrift Stores. I even taught a series of classes at my children's school about *'How to be a good friend,'* when there was a bullying problem in Charlotte's year 4 class.

I presented two papers at the Australia and New Zealand Mental Health Services conference - TheMHS - in Australia.

However, the monstrous illness that had stalked me throughout my marriage had not disappeared. Over a long period of time of ups and downs, I once again became debilitated with depression and this eating disorder i.e. symptoms of the abuse and responses to the abuse.

On several occasions, Jack told me *"You're lucky to have me. No one else would want you."* I expressed gratitude to him for this. I even repeated these words to others as if they were my own! I am gob smacked to think of this now. Firstly, that Jack would say such a thing, and secondly that I believed him and was deeply grateful!

Author Natalie Hoffman claims that we so much want to believe something, especially that a person loves us, that we only choose to see what fits with that belief, while ignoring what does not.

It was during this time that I fell deeper and deeper into depression and despair. My medication and therapy appointments increased.

She is persevering.
When she makes a commitment, she sticks to it.
Her commitment to her word is the super glue that
keeps her tied to her partner, persevering through
the confusion and pain her husband causes.
Add to this a religious community that teaches
divorce is the unforgivable sin...
and you have a very real prison from which there is no escape.
Natalie Hoffman - Is It Me?

Jack delivered messages to me that were harmful. It was hard core programming happening at my most vulnerable times. What a contrast between Dad's words in his letters, *"You are deeply loved and add value to their (Mum and Dad's) and other people's lives,"* to Jack's words — *"You're lucky to have me. No one else would want you."* Yet, I had dismissed Mum and Dad's expressed love and their gifts as disingenuous, while treating Jack as my savior. That is the power of evil and deception.

How encompassing is an abusive relationship— it dirties and destroys everything. This is an enormous overarching truth of abusive relationships.

Her religious community colludes with the abuser
by keeping the focus of her generosity disproportionately
on her since she is the active and willing partner.
This is exactly what the abuser needs to continue
harming her without experiencing any consequences.
Natalie Hoffman - Is It Me?

*****

In the period of time after the Electro Convulsive Therapy, I had an open vision that seized me. I had just gone to bed one evening and within moments, while still fully awake and looking into my darkened room, I saw four skulls cross my field of vision in slow succession. The first skull had *gaffer tape across its mouth*. The second skull had *hands covering where the ears* would be. The third skull had *protruding green spring eyeballs hanging down*. The fourth skull wore a *black hood of death*. Fear gripped me, and I was greatly shaken by this. I had not experienced anything like this before and did not understand what it meant or how to react.

I cried to Yehovah, asking Him to protect me from what felt very evil in the room. An understanding came to me that Satan was stating both his work and intention in my life. These were four demons were interfering with my communication so that I *could not speak for myself; I could not hear the Word of Yehovah; what I saw in the world around me was distorted; and they were making a pronouncement of my death.*

A Scripture verse that came to my mind was Psalm 118:17, which enabled me to combat the fear I was experiencing. ***"I will not die but live and tell what Yehovah has done!"*** I declared this verse over and over again that night and the next day, wielding it as a sword at Satan's crew. This helped keep them away from me and resist the fear.

The next day, I was still experiencing fear and still in combat with the devil with my sword. I reached out to Spirit-filled friends for prayer and counsel. I shared with them what had happened. In prayer, one of them saw Yeshua's foot come down on each skull and crush them into fine powder. Hearing this, shalom (peace) bathed my heart and mind with the reassurance that Yeshua had just destroyed the enemy's threat and plan for me. I also felt my Heavenly Father's love envelope me. Psalm 118: 17 became a ready weapon for me throughout the days, weeks and years to come, to counter the enemy's attack on my life. Sometimes I wielded *"I will not die but live and tell what Yehovah has done"* with great conviction. Other times these words were but a whisper. I believe that when suicidal thoughts prevailed and all I could manage was a whisper, it was enough to rally my angelic host to fight for me. *Death is overcome by Yeshua.* Psalm 118:17 continues to be a declaration I regularly make.

The vision I had that night was so real, that the memory of it has not faded in all these years since. It was not the only vision I would experience that would reveal my Father's heart full of love for me.

Out of my distress I called on Yehovah;
Yehovah answered me and set me free.
Psalm 118:5

There is no fear in love; but perfect love casts out fear, because fear involves torment. But he who fears has not been made perfect in love.
1 John 4:18

*****

In 2005, Jack and I were promoted to the rank of Majors, having served fifteen years as commissioned Salvation Army officers. Throughout these years, The Salvation Army had been accommodating of my poor mental health, granting me extended periods of sick leave. However, after fifteen years of yo-yo-ing health, where I would function well and then not at all, it became clear that the problem was continuing. The Salvation Army leadership asked Jack and I to consider if things might be better for me, if we were not Salvation Army officers? And so it was that later in 2005, Jack and I made the decision to resign our commissions.

We were now faced with finding our own home. To purchase a home was a tall order since we had not been salary earners. Jack had found a job with a steady income, but he realized that getting a mortgage would only be possible if we were both employed, and that my employment was that of a Registered Nurse. A bank would have confidence in my income. The problem was, I had not been working as a Registered Nurse for a good many years, my practicing certificate had therefore lapsed, and having had ECT, I was not even capable.

This did not deter Jack. I therefore needed to complete a three month 'Return to Nursing' course to gain a current practicing certificate. And so I mustered all the courage and determination I had, to do the course. It was indeed difficult for me, and to get through it was a huge accomplishment. We were then able to meet the bank's financial criteria for a mortgage, and so found a home to move into.

Once again, I was a working as a Registered Nurse, this time with a nursing agency in Wellington. I was not confident that I could manage regular work, even part-time, and so agency nursing seemed the best option for me. There were plenty of shifts available around the city since there was a shortage of Registered Nurses. This meant that I could pick and choose what shifts and where I wanted to work. Even so, my return to work as an R.N. lasted just a few short weeks. It was now well beyond my mental ability and proved to be unrealistic and hugely distressing for me.

*****

Trauma Bond

Her partner grooms her to the place where he can
offend and actually get her to feel sorry for him
because he hurt her. See what's going on here?
She not only blames herself for his mistreatment,
she feels like she failed him for not helping him enough
and actually feels sorry for what she "made" him do!
Natalie Hoffman - Is It Me?

What I did not know, and what my therapists Carmia, Chrissy and Dr. Caitlin did not know, was that a trauma bond had been established between Jack and I.

The term **trauma bonding** was developed by Dr. Patrick Carnes, and is defined as the misuse of fear, excitement, sexual feelings, and sexual physiology to entangle another person. In the 1980's, trauma bonding was used to study the effects of emotional manipulation tactics as it related to domestic abuse. Trauma bonding defines the behavior, or grooming tactics of the abuser and the resulting effect - without blaming the victim for the abuser's deceptive behavior.

As Patrick Weaver says: A trauma bond occurs in an exploitative relationship - most often an intimate relationship. The trauma bond forms subtly over time, often without the abused partner ever realizing it. The trauma bond develops from a repeated cycle of abuse and positive reinforcement. Another name for this cycle is "intermittent reinforcement," where one person gives intense affection and approval to the other person, and then alternates it with abuse, neglect, disapproval, or abandonment.

Patrick Weaver identifies these facts about trauma bonding from his website: theexodusproject.com

Fact: The Trauma Bond Is Not Love!
While a trauma bond can involve a deep emotional attachment with someone, a trauma bond is not based on love. This is because the trauma bond is not caused by love but rather by manipulation. While the victim might equate the relationship to love, the trauma bond lacks mutual care and respect. That is to say, the victim's emotions are manipulated by the diabolical behavior of the abuser whose goal is to exploit not to reciprocate genuine love. The relationship is based on deception and manipulation, which may provoke affection - but that affection is based on toxic influence, not love.

Love is patient, love is kind. It does not envy, it does not boast, it is not proud. It does not dishonor others, it is not self-seeking, it is not easily angered, it keeps no record of wrongs. Love does not delight in evil but rejoices with the truth. It always protects, always trusts, always hopes, always perseveres. (1 Corinthians 13:4-8)

Abuse, manipulation and exploitation are all behaviors diametrically opposed to what the Bible defines as love.

Fact: Trauma Bonding Is Not Just Emotional.
Dr. Elena Touroni - Chelsea Psychology Clinic, explains the effect of trauma bonding in the brain as: *"The cycle of being devalued (and then rewarded) over and over can create a strong chemical bond between the abuser and the victim. A cocktail of different hormones like oxytocin (bonding), opioids (pleasure, pain, withdrawal) and dopamine (reward) are responsible for this feeling [the victim's feelings of affection]."* When these neurochemicals are dysregulated, it can cause an emotional addiction, where a person can experience "cravings" for certain feelings or behaviors that come with the cycle.

Fact: A Trauma Bond Relationship Cannot Become Healthy.
A trauma bond relationship is not based on real love. Often, partners in a trauma bond mistake their emotional connection for real love when the feelings are a result of an abusive cycle - whether realized or unrealized. However, **trauma bonding will not turn into a healthy relationship no matter how much a person wants to believe it**.

A healthy relationship is defined by love which is respected, honored and reciprocated. A trauma bond relationship is far from mutual or genuine. It is one-sided, and while it may not appear that way at all times (in the abuse cycle), it is. It is an exploitation of emotions through manipulation and deception. Healthy emotions do not aspire or desire to be in a relationship with someone whose dysfunctional style of relating is to kill, steal and destroy the person they are with.

Fact: A Person Can Be Predisposed to a Trauma Bond.
Predisposition, however, is not synonymous with fault or victim blaming. Abusers abuse because abusers are abusers. Judas betrayed Yeshua because Judas was a betrayer (John 12:1-6), not because Yeshua made him do it. There are many historical factors that can play into our predisposition including being groomed to believe we do not deserve better, low self-esteem and fear of abandonment. Trauma bonds are

not simply like having a challenging relationship. They are deeply rooted in our basic need for attachment and security.

Fact: Prayer Alone Will Not Heal A Trauma Bond.
Deliverance is instant through faith in what is not seen, but healing takes time and work. Prayer keeps our mind focused on [Yeshua], truth and a position of authority over our struggle (Romans 5:1-5).

Fact: You Can Heal From A Trauma Bond.
Trauma is not who you are, trauma is what happened to you. The victim is not to blame for an abuser's behavior. Blaming yourself can leave you feeling more guilt and shame, which can set back your progress in moving on, and perpetuates victim blaming in abusive situations.

[End of Patrick Weaver's Comments]

*****

... if she tries to explain her experience,
the tide of that belief is too powerful to go up against.
Natalie Hoffman - Is It Me?

2024 Looking Back:
I had been prescribed a daily cocktail of anti-depressants, anti-anxiety and sleeping medications. I would wake in the morning knowing that Jack had had sex with me in the night - *while I slept!* I was conflicted about whether or not I could tell Jack that this was deeply distressing to me. However, when I finally could no longer ignore my distress, I told him that each time this happened I felt as though I had been raped. Jack was defensive and immediately retorted, *"Don't think I enjoy having sex with you when you're asleep!"* I believed that my life was a liability to Jack and sex was all I had to offer him in return. When he said he did not enjoy sex with me (in my sleep), my sense of being raped retreated, replaced by a need to placate Jack and win him

back. His words had shamed and silenced me. I was not enough. Jack continued to rape me when I was asleep.

I was not being a participant in the marriage bed for my own pleasure as it should have been. It was turned into something sick - not as Yehovah intended the marriage bed to be. Sexual violation that happens by another in our sleep when we are highly drugged and unconscious is not consensual, even if married. It is by definition - rape. It can sometimes cause worse trauma than rape by a stranger. It is a deep personal violation of trust. After all, the stranger does not come back night after night to rape his victim.

A woman who is raped by a stranger is deeply traumatized. She feels guilt, shame and vulnerability due to someone violating the boundaries of her body and home. She feels hopeless. She has wounds that take time to heal and affect her ability to have and hold relationships. Which of these issues is not made worse by a rapist and abuser that lives in her own home? Who sleeps every night in the bed beside her? And yet, the police are not going to come and take this abuser off to jail where he cannot hurt her anymore. After all, he is married to her.

Like other forms of domestic violence, marital rape is about exerting power and control over one's partner. Nearly 1 in 10 women have been raped by an intimate partner in her lifetime, including completed forced penetration, attempted forced penetration, or alcohol/drug-facilitated completed penetration. Surprisingly, rape by intimate partners is more common than stranger rape (Bachman & Saltzman, 1995; Finkelhor & Yllo, 1985; Randall & Haskell, 1995). Today the figure is higher. The United Nations International Children's Emergency Fund (UNICEF) 2024 says it is now **1 in 8 women**. The World health Organization (WHO) 2024 says **1 in 3 women**.

2024 Looking Back:
Like anorexia, psychological and sexual abuse were also spiritual battles for me that impacted me deeply. If you know of someone who is depressed or abused, it would be wise to pray and ask Yehovah for secret insight that no one else can see, so that this person can be set free from the clutches of darkness.

CHAPTER 10

Fiery Furnace

When you walk through the fire, you shall not be burned,
Nor shall the flame scorch you.
For I am Yehovah your God,
The Holy One of Israel, your Savior;
Isaiah 43:2-3

As Jack's power, control and sexual abuse continued, my mental health once again deteriorated. I was no longer able to maintain my profession as a mental health advocate. My capacity to fully parent my children decreased.

Non-Consensual & Unwanted Sexual Acts

There were many and varied unwanted sexual acts that Jack foisted upon me. When I was doing my daily tasks in the house, Jack would come up behind me and put his hand into my underwear and digitally penetrate me. This was unsolicited and unwanted. It made me feel reduced to a sex object. A *'play thing.'* Jack felt he had the right to violate my autonomy at will without my consent. The trauma bond kept me silent and confused, not knowing what to do or say about this new invasion of my boundaries. This would sometimes happen in the presence of my children when I did not feel I could protest or make a scene. I remember when Levi was doing his homework at the family PC. I was standing over him at the computer chair helping him when Jack came up from behind and penetrated me. The risk seemed to thrill him. The girls could have come in at any moment. Jack kept pushing the sexual acts further and further - seeking new thrills. I never knew what new violation would be forced upon me. **I grew hyper-vigilant. I could not sleep or even relax. A fear-reflex took over and I startled constantly at anything or anybody.**

She is forgiving.
She will overlook wrongs and forgive without being asked.
She is quick to feel bad for whatever she's done to hurt someone,
and she assumes that's how her partner feels as well.
As part of her commitment to the marriage,
and her own generous and forgiving nature,
she forgives even when the abuser isn't sorry and doesn't ask.
Natalie Hoffman - Is It Me?

*****

One day when the children were at school, Jack tied each of my wrists to either side of the bedposts using two of his neck ties. He then went off and left me. Jack thought this was funny. Me, I felt… degraded, objectified, helpless, made fun of. I felt like Jack was making a display of how things were in the relationship - he had the power to restrain and control me. I felt humiliated, yet confused that I had accepted it. What would make him think to do this to me? Why was this funny to Jack? It was a display of his power and dominance, and my submissiveness.

To control someone, is to destroy them. To control someone you have to break them down before you can reconstruct someone you can control. Jack controlling me - was Jack destroying me! I think this began subconsciously for Jack. **It was the only marriage role (the strong one and the sick one) he had ever known from his parents!** But over time his destructive actions became conscious decisions on his part, and he did them of his own free will.

I gave pieces of myself away to Jack. I loved and trusted Jack, but I was feeding pieces of myself to a monster that needed to take everything. I became mentally unwell as a consequence of Jack controlling me.

*****

I again spiraled into the clutches of anorexia, depression, anxiety and suicidality. Another hospital admission was considered necessary.

Wellington's psychiatric unit was not a good option as I had been working in the local mental health arena. So I spent about six weeks in a supervised community mental health care home in Paekākāriki, a town on the Kapiti Coast near Wellington. Here I waited for funding approval for an admission to Ashburn Clinic - a private psychiatric residential treatment program in the South Island of New Zealand.

I had been a patient there before, when it was called Ashburn Hall. It was now Ashburn Clinic. I was to discover, that it was not only the name that had changed!

While I was waiting for the funding and an admission date to Ashburn Clinic, Jack decided he wanted a collection of (pornographic) videos of me to have while I would be away from him. He had made it clear that it was a sexual sacrifice for him to allow me to go to Ashburn Clinic. He would be sexually deprived for the months I would be away. I was about to go off to a psychiatric facility for my mental illness. It was these very things that were driving me deeper and deeper into depression, and I was in a state of deep distress. At the time, I was not in any fit state to fight a battle - I was suicidal.

By claiming to be a tortured sufferer in need of relief,
a sexually abusive husband preys upon his wife's kind heart,
hoping that she'll feel sorry for him and then do what he wants.
If that doesn't work, he may escalate to using threats
while still blaming her for her own marital sexual assault.
Focus On The Family - What is Sexual Abuse in Marriage?

My boundaries had long been beaten down, so I did not consider whether or not I wanted Jack to make these videos of me, or if I would agree to let him do this. By that time, I did not have the will to say *"no."* I simply let him make these pornographic videos because he wanted it. What I did, was to feel guilty for the 'sexual sacrifice' Jack told me he would be making for me while I would be away.

2024 Looking Back:
The irrational responses, or non-responses, I had to the sexual abuse from Jack seems unbelievable to me now. I now know this is ***trauma bonding*** - it is irrational. Because of the trauma-bonding, and having had my boundaries destroyed by Jack… I let him make the videos.

This sexual filming was only of me, not Jack. It was done in two locations - our bedroom and in a hotel that Jack took me to overnight. Jack got the lingerie and outfits he wanted me to wear and told me what he wanted me doing as he filmed me. This was an all-new level of degradation for me.

Jack put the videos onto discs to watch while I was away. By the end of my time at Ashburn Clinic, I felt such shame and guilt about Jack making these videos. He had reduced me to a whore. Having been so emotionally battered, it had taken me this long for my feelings to come out, and to work up the courage to do something about it. And so I told Jack that what he had done had overstepped my boundaries in every way, and I wanted the videos and CD's destroyed. Jack responded indignantly, telling me it was his right to have them.

I was stunned. I was the only person in these pornographic videos and CD's. It absolutely was my right, and not his, to decide whether they existed or not and what was done with them! Now, I felt like my personal safety and reputation was compromised too, and by my own husband! This was deeply shocking and distressing. The man who was supposed to love and protect me, was now belligerently withholding these videos and CD's, causing me to feel extremely unsafe, vulnerable and suspicious.

Jack's argument of his 'right to the videos' made no sense to me at all. He had made these videos to have in my absence. Now I was back. Why would he not, at my request, release them to me or destroy them himself? What was his purpose in keeping them? Over-ruling my boundaries was another 'red light.' Why was he being so obstinate? Surely, he was not planning to use them as some kind of leverage over me? At the time, I could not bring myself to believe that he was capable of blackmailing me.

Abuse is fueled by entitlement

Even when we were seeing a marriage counselor together before we ultimately separated, Jack was asked multiple times by the counselor to give the videos and CD's to me. Jack would not. He remained unyielding and blatantly refused to give them over or destroy them. What was destroyed, was what little trust I had left in him.

...there is never any sowing and reaping.
Her abuser sows destruction in their relationship and in her personhood without any accountability or consequences, and she continues to forgive for the ways he causes her pain, therefore enabling the abuse cycle to continue unabated.
Natalie Hoffman - Is It Me?

2024 Looking Back:
I should not have sought to have had these marital counseling sessions with Jack to fix his abusive behavior. **Abuse is a behavioral and a public health problem, not a marriage problem** - and I was not responsible for Jack's abuse. If there was a possibility of marriage counseling for us, it should not have happened until Jack's behavior had been successfully counseled by a domestic abuse counselor.

*****

Ashburn Clinic had become a hell hole - a fiery furnace! I'd had a stint there fourteen years earlier, when it was formally called Ashburn Hall, but it had changed drastically in that time. This second admission lasted seven long, excruciating months.

Patients came to Ashburn Clinic as an alternative to state hospital care, either as private-paying individuals, or through the public health system which was funded mainly by the Ministry of Health or Accident Compensation Corporation (ACC). The ACC funding was for victims of abuse and/or trauma. While I was there, most patients were funded by the public health system. Ashburn Clinic was like a catch-all for those who were *too-hard* or *too-complex* for the other hospitals in New Zealand. These patients were vulnerable with no other suitable place to be and many were compelled to be there. This gave Ashburn Clinic a powerful upper hand, and meant these patients had to play by *Ashburn Rules* whether or not they were moral, right, fair, just, or ethical.

What Ashburn Clinic really offered was *Punishment Therapy* rather than a recovery approach! No matter what ailment brought patients there, the answer was the same - '*get a grip!*' Their treatment approach was: '*whippings will continue till morale improves!*' The process, or at least the outcome, was to punish and shame patients until they acted sane, escaped or committed suicide.

The staff at Ashburn Clinic believed themselves to be absolute truth holders. They acted as if they knew everything about a patient, and the patients knew nothing about themselves. They certainly believed that they were the experts about me!

However, there was no acceptance, understanding, or tolerance from staff of the physiological and psychological state I was in. They failed to identify the impact of domestic abuse by my husband on me. There was no recognition of the disabilities I had as a result of the Electric Shock Therapy (ECT). The ECT had injured me badly enough that I was still living with traumatic brain injury. The staff simply told me to stop annoying people by talking so slowly, and to stop crying when I was in extreme distress.

I had arrived severely depressed, underweight, highly anxious and hyper-vigilant. I was not sleeping at night. I had memory difficulties and noise sensitivity. I was halting in my speech, easily startled, and tearful. Jack had flown down to Dunedin with me, and one of the last things he said to me was, *"You can talk about about anything, but you don't talk about us!"* In my mind, there was nothing wrong with him saying this, and I was quick to agree.

Keeping family secrets is typical in abusive relationships

She is patient and long-suffering.
She will endure the attacks of her partner,
believing in his potential as a human being.
She will actively strive to endure the abuse
to the point of falling apart emotionally and physically.
Natalie Hoffman - Is It Me?

What was this cryptic message Jack was giving me? Was it normal - of no consequence? Why did I feel so compelled to exonerate Jack to everyone at every turn? He was my savior, my saint, wasn't he?

2024 Looking Back:
It seems incredible that I did not see it. Let me say it again: Jack had said, *"You can talk about anything, but you don't talk about us!"*

Jack and I had a co-dependent relationship. For things to work, I needed to be needy (sick) and he needed to be the savior. Being depressed and anxious was horrid, but my relationship with Jack was easier when I was unwell. Being well was harder in the respect that this upset the applecart of co-dependency. When I was sick he had complete control over me, and this was acceptable to me because he would apply positive reinforcement with cards of love, flowers, chocolate, special trips away for just the two of us, and other gifts.

I had no idea what was wrong. I was trying to defend Jack, but my subconscious knew there was something desperately wrong. My subconscious was pointing the finger at Jack. I was trying to submit, but my subconscious was constantly screaming at me to confront something - sometimes in irrational and unreasonable ways. It was the huge monster in the room. The sicker I got, the more desperate I became to confront this monster as a matter of survival. Confront the monster or die.

*****

As was the way with all new admissions, I was not to be in any therapy for the first week, so that I could be observed by staff. Being in a great deal of emotional distress, this meant there was no emotional support for me until my week on observation came to an end. My first small group therapy session proved to only further add to my distress.

The group was facilitated by a nurse and an Occupational Therapist. When the nurse asked me a question, I was unable to quickly respond. My brain was scrambled and I could not get my words out. The nurse was irritated by this and said, *"I don't like waiting for you to speak. You're controlling the rest of the group."* She then addressed the others in the group, *"Who else doesn't like it?"*

I was told by the nursing staff that I was not depressed, so I should stop pretending like I was. There was no response for me to make. My feelings of shame, blame and guilt were intensified. I realized that I was not going to be heard and understood. My hope of getting well… evaporated under their condemnation.

My initial one-on-one psychotherapy session did not go well either. When I knocked on the therapist's door, she opened her door for me to walk into her room. Her desk and office chair were on one side of the room, and on the other were two comfortable chairs with a small table between them. *"Please sit down,"* were her words to me. Since she had not directed me to a particular chair, I chose one of the two comfortable chairs and sat down. Just as soon as I did, she firmly questioned, *"Why did you sit there? That's my chair!"* I was shocked and taken aback! I apologized and said I did not know this. I moved to the other chair. I had not ever experienced this kind of confrontation trap used by a therapist before.

I could find no other explanation for this confrontation with her. This therapist had purposely set me up to establish her dominance, and within the first sessions it was clear that she was exerting power and control. Consequently, I failed to trust her with anything substantive. I saw this woman for fifty minutes, twice a week, for seven months, yet have no memory of her name. I compare this to the therapist I had at Ashburn Hall fourteen years earlier - fifty minutes, twice a week, for just three months - whose name was Angela and who had integrity, wisdom and kindness.

Faulty memory was one of the disabilities I continued to live with from the electric shock therapy - particularly remembering hard facts like names, places, instructions, and schedules, which were made worse under the stress and duress I was experiencing at Ashburn Clinic. This meant that I was always running to keep up with the constantly busy timetable that involved multiple meetings and therapy sessions each day, as well as community duties. It was exhausting and created a lot of anxiety for me.

To be late or missing from where we should be, was tantamount to 'disobedience' that earned the staff's reprimands and the disapproval of other patients. And so I tried as hard as I could to avoid this at all costs! I carried around with me a printed timetable which I constantly checked, as well as a notebook to keep track of things. I wrote lots of things down - things that others would easily remember - were not possible for me. Such things as people's names, what I was asked, required to do or have - the how's, where's and what's of particular house duties etc. I was told by the staff to stop doing this. They did not explain why. I presume it did not seem normal to them. But was anything 'normal' at Ashburn Clinic?

Again, it was like a set up. They required me to remember what I could not remember, so I could then be reprimanded for not remembering! It was like someone with a damaged leg needing a crutch to walk, and having them kick the crutch out from under them, and then condemning them for not being able to walk without it! I felt helpless and distressed. I was trying to get on my feet and they were pushing me back down. So I secretly carried a note book with me.

Journalling was also an important part of my life. It had helped me keep track of things and process what was going on for me. It was one of my strategies for living with the disabilities of traumatic brain injury. I would try to explain something with a verbal image or metaphor and the staff told me to stop doing this as well. I soon found out why I was told by the staff to stop journalling.

In music therapy group one day, a nurse facilitating the group shared that I had previously written a book. The nurse insinuated that I might be writing another book - a tell-all about Ashburn Clinic! She added I might be gathering writing material for such a book. She asked how the group felt about this. I can only think this was done to create distrust and suspicion of me. Someone asked me if I was going to write about them. At the time, it was not at all in my mind to write another book. Apparently, the staff were concerned I might write about them and their treatment methods. What did they have to hide? That became apparent over the following weeks and months.

As the days went on, it became clear the staff did not like how I spoke or what I spoke. They did not like how I thought or how I wrote down information. I was criticized, shamed or even disbelieved if I did not think about things in the same order, same speed, or in the same way as others. When I stopped speaking or sharing things, the staff did not like that either!

My interactions with others were often problematic to staff. If I was sitting and sharing in conversation with just one other patient, I was told I was *"colluding."* They bandied this term around constantly. Even though the meaning was somewhat vague to me, they used it as the weapon of choice with which to threaten patients. The mere accusation would strike fear into many patients. If I spent more time with certain patients and not with others, this was noticed and questioned. My friendship with other Christian patients was questioned. And as strange as this might seem, being a Christian was seen by certain staff members to be a part of my 'illness profile.' If I said something during my therapeutic sharing that related to faith, it was often met with a mocking attitude.

I was only to speak, think, process, act, and have relationships the way the staff determined for me. Anything I knew, or any skills or experience I had, were totally discounted, disregarded, or dismissed.

I saw first hand the power and control i.e. *Punishment Therapy*, being wielded by the staff over patients. The theory was to break down these troubled, vulnerable souls in order to rebuild them. Pronouncements were made over them that were often shaming, cruel and de-humanizing. These wounded individuals were further traumatized and broken. There was no 'rebuilding' apparent in staff attitudes and therapy. A nurse said in a therapy group one day, *"Not many marriages survive for those who have been patients at Ashburn Clinic."* What was hard to believe, is that such a statement would be made!

Patients were set against each other by being encouraged by staff to be judgmental of other patients. In unit and community meetings, and in therapy groups, patients were permitted to be brutally honest with their thoughts and feelings towards other patients, regardless of how damaging it might be, or however ill-informed they may be of that patient and their circumstances.

In a community meeting one morning, a young female patient sat docilely. She had decided to leave Ashburn Clinic, and the staff took turns expressing their lack of support for her decision. "*She's going off to die*," a psychiatrist expressed. I was stunned. For a psychiatrist to say such a thing is unconscionable. As a mental health professional, I had never encountered or even heard of such callous directives made to a patient by doctors, nurses or therapists - especially in the presence of other equally vulnerable patients!

Staff sometimes changed a patient's name, even against their wish, if they believed the name change would elicit different behaviors of the patient. My friend Katie was told that she would now be called Kate. She lost so much being at Ashburn Clinic i.e. home, freedom, friends, income, sport, study opportunities, and then her name was taken too!

The thing that saved me through my seven-month ordeal there, was a Christian woman named Rhonda, about my age, who lived in Dunedin and was a friend of a friend. I had never met her before, but she reached out to me as soon as I arrived in Dunedin and offered friendship. Rhonda came to Ashburn Clinic to visit me, and we quickly established a relationship. Providentially, Rhonda was a part of the *Elijah House Prayer Ministry.*

As I had not known Rhonda before this time, I had initially feared she would think I was either making things up about how rough Ashburn

Clinic was, or she would think I did not have a grip on reality. I was a psychiatric patient after all. However, this was not the case. She had already learned from an R.N. friend in her church congregation that Ashburn Clinic was not a place of righteousness, truth or healing. This R.N. had resigned her position at Ashburn Clinic after a short time, because she was so disturbed by how patients were treated.

I was allowed to go to church with Rhonda each Sunday and spend the remainder of the day at her home. While I generally only saw her on Sundays, she also supported and ministered to me in prayer throughout the weeks and months via text messages and phone calls. Throughout the seven months I was there at Ashburn Clinic, Rhonda would come before Yehovah on my behalf, either with or without me, and ask our Father questions to better understand and clarify what was truly going on. She would ask questions, then sit and listen for the answers that Father gave. Her questions were about me, Jack, my marriage, what was (spiritually) behind what was going on at Ashburn Clinic etc. She was very discerning of Yehovah's voice and careful to write down only what she heard. Anything she felt came through her own sense of things, and not from Father, she would say so. Rhonda was being more than just a lifeline to me. It was through her prayer ministry that most of my healing and restoration came. I doubt that I would have survived the harsh experience of Ashburn Clinic without Rhonda's love and prayers.

There was another R.N. (Laura) who was admitted as a patient while I was there. She was braver and more outspoken than I was. When I could only *think* about the improper treatment of patients, she would forthrightly *declare* it! Together we shared many conversations about what we saw going on, and what we thought. She was definitely seen by staff as a dissenter. The two of us together making our thoughts known was not welcome. In the very early hours one morning she was suddenly whisked away! I awoke that morning and my friend, my one source of sanity inside, was no longer a part of my life to help keep me sane. I never saw her again.

Being an R.N. myself, and having been a mental health advocate, allowed me to see things from both sides of the fence. It gave me a lens to see that what was going on was very wrong and harmful to patients.

For patients to progress and heal they need:

- An environment that fosters and supports healing and recovery. Health is not restored in an environment of threat and intimidation, dominance and control, humiliation and shaming, whether the ailment is physical, mental or spiritual.
- It is vital that patients can trust the professionals helping and supporting them. A patient cannot reasonably trust a health professional or a health system exerting power and control over them in a harmful way.
- Those administering therapy need to be responsive rather than reactive.
- There cannot be a one-size-fits-all approach when there is such variance of illness and disorder, even in a community of around sixty patients. It would be like treating everyone on a surgical ward by amputating a leg. This would not help the patient with appendicitis! What it does is make the situation worse for all patients.
- The environment must be safe and patients must feel safe. If a patient has lived through abuse or trauma - physical, sexual or verbal - that person desperately needs an environment that is not only safe but also feels safe.
- Help should be given to patients to identify and express what they already know about their condition. They will always have some degree of personal insight, and one should not ignore or discount it. Rather, the health professionals should build upon it.
- Self-respect must be maintained or recovered. Shaming patients is not ever appropriate or helpful.
- Hope and encouragement is needed for their recovery.

Ashburn Clinic failed on all accounts!

From the time of arriving at Ashburn Clinic when Jack had given me the cardinal rule: *"You can talk about about anything, but don't talk about us,"* I was being emotionally controlled by Jack. I could not question or be angry at the power and control he was using over me. For example, I could not leave Ashburn without his agreement and that of the staff. However, I was not married to the clinic staff, so I was free to question, and be angry with them for what they were doing. All the time I spent with Rhonda in prayer started waking up my Spirit to know the truth.

Patrick Weaver of *The Exodus Project* states:

When you are talking about any behavior, based on untruth,
cognitive distortion, denial, dysfunction, or destruction,
the Holy Spirit in you will sound the alarm,
your gut will sound the alarm,
and your skin will sound the alarm. Why?
For the believer, the Holy Spirit always reveals truth.
Untruth, double-mindedness, covertness, denial,
disingenuousness, or any weapon formed against you
will be revealed to you in the spirit.
The more submitted your internal truth is to the Holy Spirit,
in all things, God will reveal to you,
often in advance and in living color,
any ulterior motive or behavior that is rooted in
destruction, deception, dysfunction, untruth or evilness:

"But the Advocate, the Holy Spirit, whom the Father will send
in my name, will teach you all things and will remind
you of everything I have said to you."
John 14:26

I saw that the way staff were controlling patients was wrong. As a result of this, it became increasingly clear what was happening in my marriage. **I could see how Jack too had been controlling me and that this was also wrong.** Through the destructive power and control of staff over patients, I came to see similar tactics and outcomes of power and control in my relationship with Jack. Revelations into my life and the forces that controlled me kept hitting me like bombshells one after another. The staff were trying to control people's lives in a way that was harmful - often with tragic consequences. It became easier and easier to relate this power-lust to Jack. I eventually realized, finally, that I had to get out from under the control of Ashburn and then get out from under the control of Jack! **I started standing up and taking charge of my life.**

When I had been there several months, I witnessed a young girl who had just arrived at Ashburn. She was too young for a place like this. I welcomed her, and later asked if she would like to go for a walk on the grounds. As we walked, we briefly shared about what had brought us both here. Nikki was a vulnerable seventeen-year-old suffering with Bulimia Nervosa. It was heart-breaking to hear her story.

The next day in the morning community meeting, Nikki was exposed to the daily dose of shaming by staff and patients. In these community meetings, patients were encouraged and praised for ratting on other patients. One purpose of these community meetings was to shame and humiliate patients to 'behave better.'

This particular day, an accusation had been made by the staff that Nikki had taken someone's food from a locked freezer during the night. No evidence was given to prove the accusation true. Nonetheless, as was customary, the floor was then open to everyone and anyone to speak on the matter. It was an awful thing to witness, and I felt great pain for Nikki as she sat with her head hung low, sobbing, as she was shamed, humiliated and berated. This was the outrageous norm at Ashburn. It was the very thing that created dread in me as I walked into each community meeting. Who was it going to be today? Would it be me? Well - today it was Nikki - the young, vulnerable new girl with a life-threatening illness - who had not even been broken in to the Ashburn assault system yet!

We all knew how horrid it was to be the one with the target on their back in one of these community meetings, and so from across the far side of the gymnasium I watched intently to see if the patients sitting either side of her would offer her any support or compassion. None was forthcoming. For anyone to show compassion or speak in Nikki's defense, was to be identified as a 'colluder.' It would mean the assault would swiftly be turned on them. Who was going to invite this on themselves?

I certainly did not want to be the next target - but I stood up - and immediately I had all eyes on me. I walked across the gymnasium to Nikki with a deliberateness in my step - and handed her a wad of Kleenex that I had in my pocket. It was Kleenex that I was saving for myself in case I was the day's victim! Nikki extended her hand to take them and attempted to lift her head to look up at me. With my other hand I gently touched her knee to communicate my care, before walking back to my seat with the same deliberateness in my step. I had declared my rejection of their 'therapeutic' horror show. Subjecting someone to such ruthless shaming was dehumanizing and traumatic. It was a long walk back across the gymnasium with all the glaring eyes of the staff on me. Once sitting, I willed my body not to tremble. The heat was now off Nikki. I was now the star of the show!

"*Why did you do that?*" a staff member challenged me. It must have been Yehovah that took over from there, as I answered with a fearless clarion voice, *"I was showing her compassion!"* The patients either side of me quietly, but obvious enough to the staff, affirmed me and what I had done. And so, the whole matter was shut down in that moment. The staff said nothing more about it and moved on to another matter. That act of compassion was to rebound on me in a very personal way.

At the end of the meeting as we were all returning to our respective places, a number of patients quietly expressed their support and admiration for what I had done. "*You were so brave*," one said. How tragic that showing compassion, in this place, was an act of bravery. The staff's behavior in community meetings, as they were with Nikki, was reprehensible. How could Ashburn Clinic call itself a therapeutic community while continuing these barbaric ways? Nikki later thanked me. Mercifully, she managed to leave the next day, but how far did that experience set her back in her recovery?

Reaching out my hand to others began the process of taking charge of my life, but standing up for Nikki earned me trouble. I was told by the head nurse that what I had done in the community meeting had made staff reconsider my readiness to advance from the patient unit I was currently in, to the independent living house up the hill, in order to prepare for discharge. There, patients are allowed self-management while still in a full-time therapeutic program. This threat of-advancement was horrifying - my way out of Ashburn could be blocked! I was put through the wringer to prove I was not going to be a trouble-maker. I determined to keep my head down and my mouth shut, so I could prove myself well enough to leave. I was in survival mode, and I was fighting for my life. I also realized that in my relationship with Jack - I was fighting for my life there too.

*****

2024 Looking Back:

I had tried to quit too many times before. At this point, I decided that I would never again quit in adversity, no matter how hard, how desperate or how impossible it looked. This was a determination of spiritual significance in my life. It is what has brought me to the place of resolve where I know that **when I got knocked down, I must get back up.** Apostle Saul's declaration of faith, became mine too:

We are hard-pressed on every side, yet not crushed;
we are perplexed, but not in despair;
persecuted, but not forsaken; struck down, but not destroyed...
2 Corinthians 4:8-9

As difficult as something might be in our lives, or in the difficult days ahead, we must *always* get back up. Even when we do not know what to do, our motto must be, ***"never give up, never give in, and never quit."*** We may get knocked down, but we are not knocked out!

Do not rejoice over me, my enemy;
When I fall, I will arise; *When I sit in darkness,*
Yehovah will be a light to me.
Micah 7:8

Our enemy Satan does not have that knock-out-punch power, because as we read in 1 John 4:4, *greater is He that is in us, than he that is in the world.* Only Yehovah has knock-out-punch power!

*****

Her religious community doesn't recognize her courage,
strength, and depth of character
forged in the furnace of constant affliction.
Natalie Hoffman - Is It Me?

When a patient was getting close to their discharge date, they could expect to be thoroughly cross-examined about their readiness, plan and preparations. This would happen in various settings. It would happen with their psychiatrist or in their twice weekly one-on-one therapy time with their psychotherapist. It would also be addressed in the regular twice weekly small group therapy session conducted by one nursing staff member, a psychotherapist and six to eight patients. Then also in the the unit meeting scheduled Monday through Friday that comprised of two nursing staff, one psychotherapist, one psychiatrist, and twelve to sixteen patients, as well as in the larger community meetings scheduled Monday through Friday in the gymnasium which involved all Ashburn Clinic patients from the three units, all nursing staff, psychotherapists and psychiatrists.

This cross-examination was a harrowing experience for most, for not only did the staff challenge the patient who was looking to be discharged, but the other patients were also encouraged to challenge and express their opinions on the matter. Many a patient in my time there heard the *feared* words from staff (or other patients), *"I don't think you're ready to leave!"* Consequently, some patients buckled under the duress. When staff were unsupportive of a discharge happening, other patients might well support the staff position. Patients were discouraged from leaving, and since Ashburn was a private clinic, when patients left - revenue went with them. Leavings were a display of the staff's power and control. Patients had either a 'bad' or 'good' leaving, and there was enormous variance on how people left Ashburn Clinic.

Some left just as suddenly as they came, once they had glimpsed the Ashburn reality. These people were self-funding or not committed by the court under a Mental Health Act that required them to be there. Other 'bad' leavings, or 'escapings' I called them, were when a non-committed patient just left partway through treatment because they could not handle it anymore. Their room would suddenly be empty in the morning, and they would not turn up at the next scheduled meeting or group.

Others committed suicide to escape Ashburn Clinic. There were three suicides that I know of in 2008, around the time I was there, out of a population of some sixty patients that is an incredible 5% suicide rate! There were others who attempted suicide while I was there. I read a review from a psychologist, Dr. Suzanne Blackwell, who declared, ***"Anyone who survives Ashburn Clinic deserves a medal!"***

*****

Kayla, a beautiful young woman who I came to know at Ashburn Climic, had an eating disorder. She never got ***her medal!*** As a result of Ashburn Clinic, Kayla's life ended in tragedy. You will find her story in Appendix #1 on page 333

*****

Having a 'good' leaving depended upon whether the staff liked you or not, if the staff were supportive of the timeframe in which the patient was preparing to leave, if the staff had instigated the leaving process, and if the staff were able to maintain their control over the patient in their leaving process. Generally, the process of a 'good' leaving from Ashburn, was about four weeks. Even a 'good' leaving was tough.

Another barrier was when a patient was under a compulsory mental health treatment order. A family court judge would regularly come to Ashburn Clinic, every few weeks, to determine if these patients were ready for discharge.

One day soon after making it to the independent living house, I experienced a 'clap of thunder' that fully woke me to my reality. In that moment I realized Jack had put me, and kept me, in a sick role throughout our marriage by using the power and control which I had turned over to him. I saw how this had robbed me of my life and the life of our children. After all, it was Jack who was keeping me in this mad house. So shockingly profound was this insight that I immediately shed my sick persona. 'NO MORE!' I declared to myself. I was not sick, and I would not live this way anymore. I knew I would need to take back my personal power from Jack that I had relinquished, and he had gladly taken from me, over the years.

I once spent two weeks on a 1,000-piece jigsaw puzzle. Day by day, piece by piece, the jigsaw picture had emerged. With only a small handful of pieces left to place, there was no mystery left. There was no more wonder what the completed jigsaw picture was. The pieces in my marriage had similarly been forming a picture over the years too. Day by day, piece by piece, the jigsaw picture of me as a sick wife and mother had also been taking shape. With most of the 'pieces' placed *it was a convincing picture.* Jack had almost done it - created a whole 'jigsaw.' A picture so clear and defined, there was no wondering what the completed jigsaw picture would depict.

The nearly finished 1,000-piece jigsaw puzzle was never completed, because in a moment of intense emotional distress one day, I upended the puzzle and sent all 1,000 pieces flying! Jack had responded to me with anger when he saw me destroy the almost finished jigsaw puzzle.

And so at Ashburn Clinic that day, in a moment of great clarity and resolve, I upended the *sick-wife-and-mother-persona.* I busted up the whole picture and said, *"No more!"* I determined to no longer be a sick wife. At that moment, I sent all the pieces flying!

When a child of Yehovah knows the truth,
they are no longer dominated by the devil.

That day, I stopped taking all my medication!

Being an R.N. and having years of personal experience on psychotropic drugs, I understood the protocol of weaning off such drugs; especially those which are addictive, as two out of the three of mine were. Nonetheless I stopped all my medications cold-turkey. The only counsel I had on this was the Holy Spirit. I did not experience any side effects or withdrawal symptoms.

I had only been able to do this because I was now responsible for administering my own drugs. Rooms in the independent living house had a built-in drug lockbox and key. Prior to this transition, my drugs were administered by nursing staff who would watch to see that the drugs were taken. Once my drugs wore off I felt like a normal person who had recovered her health. I felt like I had come out of the closet into the light of the world again. I felt an enormous pride. The clinic was no place for me. I vowed I would never return here!

Having already served six months, I was desperate to leave. Clearly the staff were not the ones to assess my readiness. They had no idea what healing Yehovah was doing in me through Rhonda's ministry, while also endeavoring to combat the harm they were doing to me! Only by Divine Grace was I able to bail the water out of my boat faster than Ashburn was pouring water in!

I knew the best and quickest way to leave was to take the path of least resistance and play the game by their rules. If I did not, only Yehovah knew how long I might be imprisoned there! Even so, I would be throwing down the gauntlet the day I made my wish known to leave.

The process for discharge began in the unit meeting when a patient expressed their wish to work towards leaving. If they wanted a 'good' leaving, then they could expect the staff would want four weeks in preparation. In these four weeks, there would be much discussion with the patient about their readiness, where and with whom they intended to live, their strategies for maintaining '*good*' mental health and ongoing support etc.

You were in the minority if your leaving was supported by the staff. For most of us this was not the case. And so, it was a fearful thing to put forward a proposed leaving plan and have the plan, or timeframe, rejected or met with negativity by the staff. Even if the staff were supportive - there would be patients who were not supportive of your plan. Everyone had their say! I concluded the staff did not think patients were ever ready to leave. I suspected this had something to do with lost income from losing a patient.

My stress levels went through the roof on the day I hesitantly stated my wish to leave in four weeks' time. Sure enough there was resistance and negativity. One of the nurses had an irrational pouty response of, *"Maybe you should just leave now then!"* Another nurse said, "*You haven't got a clue what it is to be in therapy!*"

I did not respond to something so absurd. Not only had they been 'therapizing' me for five months, but I'd had many years of therapy! My mental health was not because of how I participated in therapy - it was a result of the victimization I endured. It was *these therapists who had no clue how to be therapists!* They certainly had enough clues that could have helped them to find out that the source of the problem was my husband, Jack. After all, if a woman is murdered, is not the *husband* the first suspect, even if he or others say it was not him? I had no anorexia or depression before marriage. I had developed anorexia, depression and anxiety *in* my marriage, and yet my husband was never considered as a possible cause.

We look at the parents and family circumstances of a teenager or a child who develops anorexia, but if a *grown woman* who has lived six years independently of her parents, has successfully become an R.N., has gotten married and then eighteen months later becomes anorexic, depressed and anxious… Should not the therapist be investigating the husband as the prime suspect, even if the woman and her husband say it is not him but her parent's fault? Are detectives not used to guilty people, and their family members, lying to cover up their wrongs?

Everybody missed it!

Consequently, staff did not know me or try to find out what was going on in my relationship with Jack that had put me in such a life-threatening state. Missing the heart of the matter was bad enough, but it was worse to be further abusing me in a horrendous way by their misuse of power and control. Having abused their own power to a dangerous degree - they were totally unfit and indeed unwilling - to deal with the results of abuse in their patients' lives.

Standing my ground with my plan to leave was not easy, but it was only the initial skirmish before the battle. Mostly I just stayed silent to what was said, but inside I remained resolved, and that is what counted. I dreaded every single challenge and expression of negativity that came in those following four weeks. However, knowing that an end to my Ashburn agonies was now in sight gave me hope. Nonetheless, the leaving process was not smooth sailing.

The staff took issue about Jack driving down to Dunedin to get me and having a few days together in a luxury resort. The staff badly misconstrued this and berated me about it. I told them this was Jack's plan and what he wanted. It did not matter. I was still accused of manipulating Jack to rescue me and spoil me. They determined I did not need him to drive all that way and I should just fly home.

I was caught between a rock and a hard place. Jack had made a detailed plan for a highly sexualized few days with me at a resort. He told me that he deserved this after all the months he had been without. I had the staff telling me I was putting him up to it! In their minds, this was evidence of their ill-founded belief of why I was mentally ill. All I could say was that it was Jack's idea and he wanted it this way. The staff's sniping at me continued unabated.

In my final month I met with my psychiatrist, the Director, for a clinical review. She said the staff were wondering why I did not trust them. **I stared back at her in disbelief - trying not to choke aloud at what she had just asked!** Maybe it had something to do with the fact that I had been told I knew nothing about myself, about therapy, or about what my issues really were. So I really had nothing to say. They had also told me that I did not have depression or a memory disability. There was no point saying any of this to the psychiatrist! So I said nothing - rather than take the risk of sabotaging my release.

Patients, independent of the staff, would plan a farewell party for someone leaving Ashburn. This occasion was free of staff members and typically was a really lovely relaxed and fun time, as was my own farewell party.

Patients were also given opportunity to say goodbye throughout someone's final week, in each of the group sessions. All the patients expressed words of love, support and appreciation to me. This seemed to be a bitter pill for the staff to swallow. There were many positive things said to me by patients that the staff immediately tried to shoot down. In my last small group therapy session, the psychotherapist shot a final arrow at me saying, *"You'll be back here!"* Such an unprofessional comment was shocking. It only served to make me more resolute. I was getting out of Ashburn and **never** coming back!

I made my *declaration of independence* in art therapy the day before being released from Ashburn. The head nurse asked us to draw or paint something on a particular therapeutic topic. We would then tell the group about it - each of the group members and staff would make comments. Today I was feeling emboldened, because at this point, I had nothing to lose. My release date and arrangements were final so there was not anything staff could do to threaten my leaving. I worked on my sheet of paper with unusual freedom. It no longer mattered how staff or patients might respond when my turn came to explain the 'what' and 'why' of my art.

I am no artist by any means, but today I took the clear strong images I had in my head and depicted them with equally clear strong strokes on paper, surprising even myself! On one side of the paper, I drew a sad, broken house with broken windows and door, and thunder clouds above. The lines were vague and uncertain. The color was predominantly black. On the other side I drew the same house, but now it was clean, cleared, restored to vibrant colors. This time the lines were strong and definitive. The sun was shining. These two images depicted what I had been, and what I now was. I felt very clear about my life. I had broken free from my ruins, and from this fiery furnace called Ashburn Clinic.

When it came my turn to hold up my paper and explain, I did so with unusual calm and strength. I had no fear of the feedback or the questions I might be asked. The nurse expressed surprise, "*This is different. I haven't seen this side of you before.*" I responded, "*There is a lot about me that you don't know.*" She invited further comment, so I did not hold back. I told her and the group that this place had not permitted me to be open or real. I had tried to be both but was rebuked or diminished for it. I had therefore found wellness despite things at Ashburn. The nurse really had nothing to say. The patients were shocked at my boldness.

Fiery Furnace

Yehovah hates injustice and grieves with those who suffer abuse. He did not intend for us to experience the terrible pain of trauma. But even in the darkest moments, when we have felt abandoned by Yehovah, He has promised to be with us.

As Psalm 23:4 says, *"Even though I walk through the valley of the shadow of death, I will fear no evil, for you are with me."* Yehovah was right there in the midst of my suffering, even when I could not perceive His presence.

In Daniel 3:8-25 there is a story of Shadrach, Meshach and Abednego. They would not bow down and worship King Nebuchadnezzer and so faced punishment of death by a being thrown into a fiery furnace. They had told the king, *"Our God whom we serve is able to deliver us from the burning fiery furnace, and he will deliver us out of your hand, O king."* (Daniel 3:17)

In a fiery furnace that should have cooked them to a crisp, they did not get consumed. In fact, they walked out unaffected from the fire because Yehovah-Yeshua was the forth man, supernaturally, in the fire with them. Their lives were therefore preserved!

Yehovah did not save them from
being **put in the fire**,
He saved them **in the *midst* of the fire**.
They came out not even smelling of smoke!

Just think, if you or I sat around a campfire, we would smell of smoke, but there was no evidence of their ordeal, not even the smell of smoke on them! Praise Yehovah!

Since Yehovah is the same yesterday, today and forever, and He is no respecter of persons, then if He did this for Shadrach, Meshach and Abednego, He can and will save us from our fiery furnaces! Remember, Yeshua is Immanuel, meaning, ***"God with us."*** (Matthew 1:23)

Yehovah-Yeshua showed up in the middle of their trauma and walked with Shadrach, Meshach and Abednego through it. In the same way, no matter what abuse, trouble or persecution we experience, Yehovah is with us. He loves us and promises to be with us through every 'fiery furnace' experience we go through. He **can** and **will** bring us out without even smelling of 'smoke.'

*****

One might expect that after seven months in a health treatment facility, a person finally well enough to leave would have an overflow of gratitude to the staff for their help. There would be mutual heartfelt goodbyes and well-wishes from staff. My experience at Ashburn had not produced gratitude. It had produced quite the opposite. No staff member had anything positive to say, only perfunctory goodbyes.

When I left Dunedin, Rhonda gave me a card with these words she had heard from Yehovah for me:

You have a race to run that's not finished yet.
There is more in this life to experience and express.
With the choosing of life each day, you are choosing Me!
For where I AM, hope dwells and thrives.
In Me, daughter, you will soar to heights you have not known.
The lows, as you have known them,
will go, but not go completely.
Don't fear them.
It doesn't matter where you are, I AM with you.
Heights and depths present no difficulty to Me.
Remember: Where I AM, hope dwells and thrives.
And, I AM with you."

*****

Healing Prayer:
Father Yehovah, we lift up the Ashburn Clinic and all clinics that are like it. Yeshua taught us to love our enemies and pray for those who persecute us. We ask you, Father, forgive all of the wickedness that goes on in these clinics, and place the blood of Yeshua on every single person that works at these clinics and every single person that is a patient. We ask You, Father, to set every abuser free from all the forces of wickedness that operate through them. We bind every spirit of darkness and paralyze their works and effects. We destroy the works of the enemy who tries to steal, kill and destroy these precious ones who are suffering.

We also ask that You strengthen every patient and help them see the truth and know You are near. We thank you for those of Your children who came alongside me to give me hope and courage and prayer support. May every patient of these clinics be blessed with someone of great faith as well, so they are able to break free from all bondages.

We ask that every clinic that does not operate in Your love and light be exposed and shut down. May Your powerful love bring healing and wholeness to all humanity.

In the mighty name of Yeshua, we pray, Amen.

Dear friends, don't be surprised or shocked that you are
going through testing that is like walking through fire.
Be glad for the chance to suffer as Christ suffered.
It will prepare you for even greater happiness
when he makes his glorious return.
1 Peter 4:12-13, CEV

The Exodus

And Yehovah spoke to Moses, "Go to Pharaoh and say to him,
'Thus says Yehovah ***"Let My people go, that they may serve Me…"***
Exodus 8:1

CHAPTER 11

Red Sea Road

But when Pharaoh saw that there was relief, he hardened his heart and did not heed them, as Yehovah had said.
Exodus 8:15

Jack worked hard to get me into Ashburn and then to keep me there for what seemed an indeterminant length of time. I had agreed to the admission, but I had no idea it would mean seven months of abuse, or that I would not be allowed to leave. Jack took power over my life. I had described to him in detail the hell hole that Ashburn had become. Jack knew what he was putting me through. I very quickly realized I did not want to be there at all. It was toxic to my mental health. Rather than get me out, I was kept there for seven months. When I had expressed to Jack my intention to work towards discharge, he countered -

"It's not up to you when you leave. It's up to me and the staff."

This was the *first* big red warning light!

The discharge conference call had taken place between me, Jack, the head nurse and another staff member. During this call, Jack repeated the incredible statement he had made so often spoken during our lives together:

"Cate being well will be like her shooting off into space like a rocket ship, and I will be left as the unwanted and abandoned launch pad."

That was the *second* big red warning light!

I refuted this and told him I just wanted to be well. Amazingly, Jack's revealing remark did not raise any eyebrows among the nursing staff, nor elicit any comment from either of them. Maybe it was not so amazing since the head nurse had previously stated that, ***"Not many marriages survive for those who have been patients at Ashburn Clinic."***

The day I was to leave, Jack arrived and parked the car in the carpark next to the building where I had been living for the past months. He knew the patient daily schedule, and that I would be walking back to this building at lunchtime. He was lounging across the hood of the car. I realized that Jack was posing himself, perhaps as my *'knight in shining armor'* coming to save me! It was a little late for that.

That evening Jack and I got to the luxury resort suite. I was thoroughly exhausted by my ordeal at Ashburn Clinic and enormously relieved at my release. Jack had a good bottle of wine, my sexualized black prostitute outfit, and an eager expectant look on his face. I put my head on the pillow and slept. So much for Jack's plan for a hyper sexualized getaway.

In that moment Jack's dominance over me melted away!

With each cycle of illness it had been harder and harder to claw my way back up out of the pit to health. I never wanted to go back to the hospital - the children needed me alive and well. *I* needed me alive and well!

She willingly sacrifices, believing that it is worth it
if he will one day finally recognize what he is doing to her
and stop and become the
good man she believes he can be....
This plays into her partner's agenda to keep her
doing what he wants her to do—all in the name of God.
This is ultimate spiritual abuse.
Natalie Hoffman - *Is It Me?*

The day after we got home from my time at Ashburn Clinic, Jack and I were outside in the garden. I said to him: ***"Jack, if I ever have to make the choice between being well and being in relationship with you, I need to choose to be well."***

I knew these were very sobering words for Jack to hear, but I anticipated him saying something like, *"well.... let's make sure you will never have to make that choice."* Instead he angrily retorted,

"This is not a decision you can just make by yourself!"

I was dumbfounded. I had envisioned us being able to have a successful relationship at last - now that we could be equally healthy.

That was the *third* big red warning light!

Jack's knee-jerk reaction confirmed for me the damaging effects of his power and control over me. It was the final big red warning light that catalyzed me to throw off his power and control. I was not threatening or planning to leave him. Nonetheless, Jack's response cut me like a knife. I was trying to explain that I could never go into that darkness again, no matter what I had to do. When he said that - it became even more clear that Jack did not want me to be healthy.

I realized that Jack was not capable of changing the dance step we had danced together throughout our marriage. Jack saw this as me turning the table on him. He took it hard. He was confounded, morose, and angry.

A short time before I had been admitted to Ashburn Clinic, Jack had said something that seemed very strange to me at the time. He said, ***"If we ever break up, you would easily remarry. No one would want to marry me!"*** Now it all came into sharp focus and made sense. At first, Jack had probably subconsciously carried over the pattern of sick dependency from his parents' relationship. However, for a long time now Jack had been consciously choosing to keep me sick out of a fear of abandonment. He saw my health as a threat, in that if I was well, I would leave him, believing that no woman would want him if she were well and strong.

She is courageous.
She survives the rejection of her love
and dehumanization of her spirit,
and still she goes into each day with hope.
Her courage in the face of daily abuse,
both covert and overt, is incredible.
This inner strength is exploited by her abuser
who is both jealous of her
strength and desires to use it against her.
Natalie Hoffman - Is It Me?

*****

Returning from Ashburn Clinic, I had reestablished my personal boundaries with Jack. One of these boundaries was around sexual intimacy. I was now clear in my own mind about what was and was not okay for me sexually with Jack, and of not being coerced into perverse sexual behaviors.

Jack had made it clear to me in the later years of our marriage, that my only redeeming value to him, was my ability to sexually service him. While I had once believed this, I no longer believed it to be true, and I no longer wanted to experience sex with Jack in the same way we once had. I no longer wanted to dress up for him, role-play 'Candy,' or have sex when I did not want to. Instead, I desired normal-loving-sexual-intimacy with Jack. Such a 'down-grade' was displeasing to Jack and provoked his anger. For him, I was denying him his sexual entitlement to me.

Sexually abusive oppressors
believe that they are entitled to sex.
These husbands genuinely feel entitled to their spouse's body.
They love themselves and their own pleasure to such an extent
that they will harm another person to satisfy themselves.
Focus On The Family - What is Sexual Abuse in Marriage?

I remember several conversations with Jack, in response to this 'down-grade.' One related to chocolate! Jack had come to compare my need for chocolate, to his need for sex. I do not know how long this was the case, but it became apparent sometime after I had returned home from Ashburn Clinic. He became jealous that I could buy chocolate to satisfy my craving, while he saw me as denying his craving (for sex). One day he said to me in a grieved tone, *"It's hardly fair that you can buy chocolate when I can't buy sex."*

2024 Looking Back:
I was refusing to satisfy his addiction to sex.

Another conversation was when Jack and I were in the city one night. It was just us; the children were at home. In the dark of night, Jack was driving us home through the city and past a brothel. He pointed to the flashing neon lights of the establishment, and in a cool and condemning tone said to me, *"If I fall into temptation, you will be responsible!"* I was made speechless by the impact of those words, saying nothing as he drove us home. I now wonder if he already had *'fallen into temptation.'* What about all those nights he did not return from work until the children were already in bed?

Once when Jack was very unhappy with me, I asked him what he was upset about. He said it was, *"your lack of interest in my body."* I told Jack I was sorry he was feeling this way and explained that his loving emotional connectedness to me would be the key, something that was not happening. This agitated Jack. He said I was making excuses, and that if his body did not turn me on, he would go out and find women who were turned on by his body. **I later learned that these are common threats from sexual abusers.**

It is not a wife's job to keep her husband from sin.
Each person is responsible for his or her own sin.
(see Luke 6:45)

Throughout the twenty-two years of marriage to Jack, it was difficult for me to recognize that I was being sexually abused, because I was married to him. How can that be abuse?

2024 Looking Back:
The signs of this abuse were clear: coercion or manipulation to

engage in unwanted sex acts, lack of consent, fear and anxiety around sexual interactions, feeling ashamed and guilty about sexual experiences.

Every cell in our body has memory. Every cell in our body can feel the violation of doing, seeing, acting in ways that are not wanted. It was no wonder I had anorexia. My body was in revolt! **If I was not going to be treated as a woman who is loved, then I was not going to eat.** It was only my relationship with Yehovah that saved me through this ordeal.

Your gut and your instincts will always feel
the effect of maltreatment because
maltreatment is an act of aggression.
For an abuse victim, bad behavior is not an event,
it is a pattern of diabolical, manipulative, untruthful,
and negative behavior unrelated to you and is rooted
in their dysfunction — that activates
your body's fight, flight, freeze, or fawn response.
Patrick Weaver - The Exodus Project

It was during the seven long months in a psychiatric clinic at the other end of the country - separated from my children and home - that I came to realize the damaging effects of Jack's power and control over me.

I had to take back my personal power from Jack that he had taken from me over the years. I had to reestablish normal healthy boundaries with him. I had to change the *dance step* in our relationship. I thought and hoped that Jack would see this as a good thing! My overwhelming desire was for a healthy marriage with Jack. It would now be different. We would be equals, striving and thriving together.

For the next eighteen months I was completely medication free, clear minded, fully and lovingly engaged with the children and with life. I was no longer a 'sick' wife, and I was reestablishing normal healthy boundaries with Jack. Though I still had challenges remaining from the ECT, I was the most well, and functioning, I had ever been in my married life. For Jack, he had lost his power and control over me. This provoked great anger - anger that he projected on me.

Jack would leave the house for work each day very early before the children were up and arrive home after the children were in bed. I picked up the tasks of parenting and household tasks with ease and diligence. On the weekends when Jack was not at work, he was withdrawn and morose, moving around the house wearing a hoodie over his head. I did my best to engage Jack in positive ways, but as Jack was collapsing, our marriage too was being collapsed.

*****

We did get marriage counseling, despite Jack's reluctance. At one of these sessions, we talked about personal boundaries. I stated that I felt profoundly unsafe and demeaned by the sex toys and erotica Jack had for many years wanted me to wear and use. I also asked in no uncertain terms that Jack return the sexual videos he had made of me - a request that he had been resisting. Jack once again insisted he needed the videos and that it was his right to have them.

At the time that he made these videos, my thinking was still so sick that I was unable to stop him - even though I knew it was wrong and degrading. Now, the *well* me definitely wanted them destroyed. The counselor strongly supported my right to do so. Jack refused to give them up. The photos and videos were about Jack's power and control over me.

Only in hindsight did I realize that these attempts at marriage counseling were not wise. They made a bad situation worse. Again, to be clear - **Jack's abuse was a behavioral problem not a marriage problem. I was not responsible for his abuse.**

*****

There were times of physical threat towards me and the children. Once Jack, in a rage, punched his fist clear through the kitchen wall in front of the children and I.

An abuser is always good to you until they're not...
The motive behind their behavior may never and doesn't
need to be known in order to know they are abusive.
What is observable is their behavior.
The Holy Spirit will always reveal, predict,
and give you a complete picture of the truth about behavior
when it is against you, and when it's motivated by evil
or negativity... pay attention (see Matthew 26:17-25).
Patrick Weaver - The Exodus Project

Another time, Jack became enraged in a marriage counseling session with me, facilitated by a Catholic priest. Jack angrily rose from his chair and exploded. He paced around the small room, violently shredding a Kleenex box until it was completely destroyed, while swearing obscenities at the top of his voice! It was scary! The priest did nothing to stop him or calm him. I think the priest was shocked. He just stared at Jack and eventually addressed me, asking if I was aware that Jack was this angry. All I could do was nod affirmatively. I had to drive home with Jack in a state of rage. I was terrified!

There were nights when Jack would come to bed in that same seething state of rage! I would be in the bed, when he would come into the bedroom tense and brisk. It was like a white anger exuding from him that I could feel. He would not speak to me in this intense state, nor would I speak to him. I was petrified! When Jack got into bed with me like this, I huddled on the edge of the bed as far away from him as I could be. I had no idea what he might do to me. I remained hyper-vigilant, while pretending to be asleep.

When Jack could contain himself no longer in the bed, he would burst out in a fury and take himself to the veranda outside our room. There he would be for a time before returning to the bedroom. All the while, stoking his anger, making a show of it. He was causing me to live in fear, with the implied threat that he could lose it at any moment. His anger was a weapon of control. **He was not trying to control it. He was using it to control me.** It kept me afraid the whole time.

When he returned to bed, I stayed awake till I heard him sleeping. My heart was in my mouth. There were repeated nights for me like this when I started to resist his power and control over me.

Abusers don't **not** *want to abuse.*
Their intent is always to abuse.
That is what their goal is.
Everything is towards that goal of abuse.
Kim Olden, M.Ed., LPC-S - Director of Trauma Services

Another episode of Jack's rage and physical violence was with Levi. Levi was 10 years-old at the time and had said something Jack did not like. Instantly, Jack grabbed Levi by his shoulders and pinned him up against a wall, angrily venting at him. Levi was terrified, as was I!

I screamed at Jack to put him down! He did. Levi ran at top speed up the stairs to his bedroom sobbing. I had not seen Jack lose his temper so badly with any of the children before. With me, yes, but *not* the children. That was the last straw for me!

*****

Moreover, I have heard the groaning of the people of Isra'el,
whom the Egyptians are keeping in slavery;
and I have remembered my covenant.

"Therefore, say to the people of Isra'el: ***'I am Yehovah.***
I will free you from the forced labor of the Egyptians,
rescue you from their oppression,
and redeem you with an outstretched arm
and with great judgments.

I will take you as my people, and I will be your God.
Then you will know that I am Adonai your God,
who freed you from the forced labor of the Egyptians.
I will bring you into the land which I swore to give to Avraham,
Yitz'chak and Ya'akov — I will give it to you as your inheritance.
I am Yehovah.'"
Exodus 6:5-8 (CJB)

I began my relationship with Jack being a fully functioning and competent adult. Then I abandoned my boundaries and gave over my personal power to him, not knowing the unimaginably tragic consequences. It took more than twenty years of marriage, but I finally came to understand what was happening in my relationship with Jack that kept me perpetually cycling between life and death. I was an adult again with my boundaries reestablished and having taken back my personal power. Jack was no longer controlling me. I was not a victim anymore. I had totally shed my victimhood.

When I left Ashburn Clinic, I walked away from Anorexia Nervosa, and the depression that came with it, like it had never consumed me! It was as if the six hospitalizations, the four suicide attempts, the endless psychotherapy, and blaming my parents - had never happened.

I dove back into being a loving daughter and mother tending to three active children and all their school and extra-circular activities. I was not like the girl I used to be, but I was free of the affliction and full of energy and joy. My eating and weight returned to normal. **I have never had a problem with anorexia again!**

*****

On average, it takes a woman seven attempts
to leave an abusive relationship for good.
Jane Clayborne, Community Relations Director
James House - Shelter for Victims of Domestic Violence

Interestingly as I look back, I also had multiple 'exit' attempts to leave my relationship with Jack and the Cruel Master - Satan. This was *not* by physically packing my bags and leaving Jack. It was rather by being so depressed I gave up on life! It was by attempting suicide and requiring hospital admissions. I am able to count up six of these specific occasions, before I finally separated from Jack - with my life! - on the seventh. This happened with the help of the Wellington Women's Refuge Services.

I came to realize that the 'truth' had been manufactured by Jack and force-fed to me throughout our marriage. Although there were still months of revelation and confrontation ahead of me - I now had the clarity to see everything in it's proper context. I had cut to the core of the problem after so many years of life-threatening mental illness. I was rapidly realizing the real truth ever more clearly. There were still battles left to fight, but the war had reached a turning point. Somewhere, somehow my spirit subconsciously led the way in what I had to do. My conscious mind hustled to keep up. But by now I had separated myself from Jack's control and the toxic programing that came with it. Satan had tried to take me out and he had failed!

*****

The Israelites were slaves in Egypt, though they had begun their sojourn in Egypt as a healthy, thriving people group. Then came a new Pharaoh who severely oppressed and harshly treated the Israelites - even having them beaten by their cruel taskmasters. They experienced extreme bondage. In time, the Pharaoh came to perceive the Israelites as a potential threat to his power and authority as they grew is strength and numbers. He therefore tried to suppress and control the growing Israelite population by ordering the midwives to kill all newborn Israelite baby boys and throw them in the river Nile!

Similarly, I began my life as a healthy and thriving individual too. Then came a toxic husband and the Cruel Master of anorexia where I too experienced extreme bondage. When I was growing in health and strength - mentally, physically, and spiritually after coming back from Ashburn Clinic - I was perceived by Jack as a threat to his power and control in our relationship, and to the status quo of our relationship.

But we have this treasure in earthen vessels,
that the excellence of the power may be of God and not of us.
We are hard-pressed on every side, yet not crushed;
we are perplexed, but not in despair; persecuted,
but not forsaken; struck down, but not destroyed -
2 Corinthians 4:7-9

2024 Looking Back:
The reader may find that the source of my mental illness was quite clear. It is to me now, as well. So why could I not see it during all those years of desperate pain and suffering while in the grip of the life-threatening disease of anorexia? I was like the Israelites in Egypt under Pharaoh's rule and control. Their slavery had become a normalized reality for them. This was all they knew. Then Yehovah came to their rescue.

Somewhere in my subconscious I knew that to see the truth might well cost me my husband and family. It was that reality which caused me to deny the elephant in the room - that Jack needed to subjugate me just as Pharaoh needed to subjugate the Israelite slaves.

The Exodus - Leaving Egypt

And Yehovah spoke to Moses, "Go to Pharaoh and say to him,
'Thus says Yehovah
"Let My people go, that they may serve Me…" ' "
Exodus 8:1

Just as Moses was instructed to confront Pharaoh, Yehovah helped me muster the courage to confront Jack. I told Jack we needed to separate so he could sort out his anger as it was putting us all at risk. I told Jack he would have to leave, and I would care for the children. And just like Pharaoh, Jack resisted this, but I did not back down. And so because I was not seeking a permanent separation - I was not clear enough or courageous enough about that! - Jack left the family home two months later on April Fool's day, the 1st of April of 2010. Our children remained in my care.

So Pharaoh said, "I will let you go, that you may sacrifice to
Yehovah your God in the wilderness;
only you shall not go very far away. *Intercede for me.*
Exodus 8:28

*****

There are various reasons why women are reluctant, or struggle, to leave an abusive relationship. And I imagine the Israelites would have shared some, if not all, of these very same reasons:

- Emotional and psychological manipulation
- Financial dependence
- Lack of resources (e.g., alternate housing, income)
- Isolation from friends and family
- Fear of violence or retaliation
- Cultural or societal pressures that discourage leaving
- Disability or other vulnerabilities that make it harder to escape

The messages that kept whirling around in my head were:

- *Jack won't allow it. He'll get angrier with me.*
- *Jack is right. I will never make it on my own.*
- *I am not financially independent.*
- *I have no income.*
- *No one in my family has ever separated or divorced.*
- *It's "wrong."*
- *My family won't understand.*
- *People will think I am bad.*
- *I am not equipped to deal with all this...*

When I consider the Israelites' bondage under Pharaoh in Egypt, how different were my fears and thinking to that of theirs? When Moses had them getting ready for escape, they would have had thoughts like:

- *Isn't this just our lot?*
- *But this is all we have ever known!*
- *Where will we go? It's too scary!*
- *But we're dependent on Pharaoh!*
- *We'll have no food or houses...*
- *Who will protect us?*
- *Pharaoh and his army will come after us! We'll be done for!*

These reasons and fears did not stop the Israelites leaving under Yehovah's guidance and Sovereign mighty hand. These reasons and fears did not stop me either. I too permanently separated from Jack under Yehovah's guidance and Sovereign mighty hand. Moses gave the Divine instructions to the people as to what the Israelites should do to prepare. I too was Divinely instructed. Was it easy for the Israelites? No. Was it easy for me? No.

So the heart of Pharaoh was hard; neither would he let the children of Israel go, *as Yehovah had spoken by Moses.*
Exodus 9:35

Jack, like Pharaoh, had *not* been willing to let me go either. He was also determined that if he could not have me, he would go to extreme lengths to make sure that *no one* wanted me - *including our children.* Jack had also made a threatening parting shot to me when we separated:

"If you ever write about this,
I will make your life miserable.
I will sue you!"
- Jack

For the following two years I contended with Jack in the Family Court, attempting to rescue my children from the brain-washing that Jack was doing to them. He had declared me to be an unfit mother, and that I was putting our children at physical and psychological risk. He proceeded then to turn the children against me in despicable ways. This two-year long experience was an excruciating, heart-breaking and devastating time for me. The children became as hostile toward me as their father had become. Jack ensured that my rights and responsibilities to be a mother to our children were stripped from me. This was not at the decree of the impotent Family Court, but by Jack's cruel design and deceptions. I will write more about these two years in my following book, ***A Voice in the Wilderness.***

When the New Zealand mandatory two-year wait time before filing for a divorce was up, Jack served me divorce papers. This he did exactly two years to the very day of our legal separation. As I consider the Exodus story, Jack serving divorce papers on me was like Pharaoh sending the Israelites out of the land after the tenth severe plague had struck the Egyptians (Exodus 12:29).

Divorce can be a gift of God's mercy for abuse victims.
Natalie Hoffman - flyingfreenow.com

The Israelites left Egypt in a state of urgency, with little time to prepare or gather extensive possessions. They were forced to flee with only what they could carry, including their kneading bowls, cloaks, and staffs, as well as some hastily baked unleavened bread (Exodus 12:39).

Similarly, just weeks after the final court hearing I'd had a couple of friends help me sell everything I had, so I could buy a plane ticket out of New Zealand. I was deeply traumatized, and if there was to be any hope of survival for me - emotional and physical - I needed to leave and leave quickly. And like the Israelites fleeing Goshen, I too fled New Zealand with only what I could carry - two suitcases.

I would have lost heart, unless I had believed
That I would see the goodness of Yehovah
In the land of the living.
Wait on Yehovah; Be of good courage,
And He shall strengthen your heart;
Wait, I say, on Yehovah!
Psalm 27:13-14

When the Israelites were faced with an impossible situation with an Egyptian army behind them and the ocean in front of them, Yehovah told Moses to tell the people, *"Yehovah will fight for you; you need only to be still."* (Exodus 14:14) Yehovah then opened the mighty Red Sea, making a way where there had been no way. And at this point, the Israelites surely had thought, *"Imminent death is behind us and we are definitely going to die if we stay here, but to trust Yehovah and walk through the middle of an ocean is terrifying! That may kill us as well!"*

As I waited to board my plane at Wellington's airport in November of 2012, about to leave the only homeland I had ever known, I felt like I was standing on the very edge of the highest Olympic diving board… in the darkness of night…about to jump - yet not knowing if there was even any water in the diving pool! I had no idea what lay ahead. All I could do was trust that Yehovah would *part the waves and deliver me.*

This was my ***Red Sea Road*** that took me on a search for the ***'Promised Land'.***

Thus says Yehovah, who makes a way in the sea,
And a path through the mighty waters,

Who brings forth the chariot and horse,
The army and the power
(They shall lie down together, they shall not rise;
They are extinguished, they are quenched like a wick):

"Do not remember the former things,
Nor consider the things of old.
Behold, I will do a new thing,
Now it shall spring forth;
Shall you not know it?

I will even make a road in the wilderness
And rivers in the desert."
Isaiah 43:16-19

The Israelites of the Exodus were yet destined to go to Mount Sinai - *the Mountain of God.* Although I did not know it… so was I! We both had an appointment with Yehovah at His Holy Mountain.

13 years later… I am living in Texas, USA

Please note: In my following book,
A Voice in the Wilderness,
the story of my 12 years in the *wilderness* is told.
See Preview page 348

CHAPTER 12

Marriage at Mount Sinai

You in Your mercy have led forth
The people whom You have redeemed;
You have guided them in Your strength
To Your holy habitation.
Exodus 15:13

I became a believer in the significance of celestial events in the Heavens on March 14, 2023 when I was remarried at the base of Mount Sinai in Midian. **The miracles - celestial events - that were unleashed after the Ketubah ceremony will be forever fixed in my memory!** The Ketubah was a marriage covenant between Yehovah and His chosen people which is outlined in chapter 19 of Exodus and the succeeding chapters. It would be 3,500 years before the Ketubah ceremony would be re-enacted at Mount Sinai - and the only time ever done there by a New Covenant group of believers. However, this part of the story did not start there, and it is a story that does not end there. Of that, I am certain!

As it has been said, time is thought to be cyclical in some Eastern cultures, while in the West we see it more as linear. But could it be both? We often see events - even fulfillment of prophecy - being repeated throughout history on different levels, as if using the same template. The bottom line is that our Creator has a masterplan, and history is unfolding His great redemptive plan. We are not to fear the future because Yehovah, the One who made time, has given us the Scriptures describing the beginning, the middle and the end. This helps us understand the times and seasons we are in. Yehovah has already prepared the footsteps of our lives. Every single one of them is known to Him, and His timing is precise and calculated. Of this, I am also certain!

For two decades, Dr. Jones had been researching the earliest alphabets on stone, tracing their origin to Arabia and the Exodus. His book, *Writing of God: The Secret of the Real Mount Sinai*, documents these findings. In October of 2022 he was asked to partner with Living Passages, a travel company, and lead a tour to the Mountain of God, called Jabal al-Lawz, Mount Sinai, and the surrounding areas in Midian. The tour was scheduled for March of 2023. Tourism in the Kingdom of Saudi Arabia was, and still is, in its infancy - but with the ever-increasing political stability of the region – the northwest corner of Arabia has begun to divulge its buried secrets.

Dr. Jones asked me if I would like to go on this tour and research expedition. Of course I wanted to go to the real Mount Sinai! This journey would give the opportunity for Dr. Jones and his team, including me, to study the land, inspect the evidence and document it. We would be in the genuine locations as depicted in ancient manuscripts and see antiquities that had remained behind the veil. So I asked Yehovah if I could go on this journey to His holy mountain - Har Yehovah. I asked if this was in His plan for me. At this time, Dr. Jones and I were engaged with no wedding date set.

I had met Dr. Jones in Kerrville, Texas in the USA one summer evening of March 2020 while at a friend's birthday party. This was just days before Dr. Jones had been scheduled to go to New Zealand and Australia on a book tour. It was also at the time of the Covid plandemic and the governments of both these countries had just closed their borders to non-citizens. So only days before Dr. Jones was to have left for New Zealand he happened to meet me, a New Zealand woman in the beautiful garden of a local restaurant where I was walking my dog.

On my part, I was not seeking to exchange anything more than a courteous greeting, yet Dr. Jones clearly wanted to talk. He had deciphered my non-Texan accent as either New Zealand or Australian and had thought - "*Wow... if I can't go to New Zealand, then Yehovah has brought New Zealand to me!*"

As I attempted to politely end the conversation, Dr. Jones told me he was an author and had been about to go to New Zealand and Australia on a book tour. A likely story I thought! But what a great way to impress! I felt obliged to ask, "So w*hat do you write about?*"

"*Religious topics*," was his response. Hmmm. I could have stopped there, but I could see he wanted me to ask him, *"what religious topics?"*

"What kind of religious topics?" I asked.

"The real Mount Sinai, the writing of God, education..."

He did not have a business card to give me, but he had told me his name was Dr. Miles Jones. Okay, so I could look him up online and see if he was for real or not.

He continued by asking what brought me to Texas? I answered nonspecifically, "*I go where God leads me*." He asked me what kind of work I did. I told him I was a seamstress. Feeling somewhat undone having this man ask more questions than I felt comfortable to answer, he asked if I had a business card. I gave him one and said goodnight.

Once home, I looked for him online and found he was indeed the Dr. Miles Jones of his claims, and that Benai Emunah (meaning *household of faith*) was the name of his institute. I was even intrigued about what he apparently wrote and taught about. I did not expect he would call me the next day and tell me he had a jacket that needed repairing. Well, maybe I did! He asked if he could buy me lunch at the same restaurant where we had met, so he could bring me the jacket. Smooth move! I found myself saying yes to Dr. Jones, and so we met once more in the beautiful garden of the restaurant.

Sitting at a table under a sun umbrella eating a delicious salad, he spoke about the earliest writing being the "writing of God" in Exodus 32:16, and of where he had discovered T*he Hebrew Gospels* that were not supposed to exist. He also told me that Yeshua was Jesus' actual name and that God's real name was Yehovah. He told me that while Jesus and Yeshua were the same historical person, they had different archetypes. He told me things that I had not known - and I had questions for everything he was telling me.

Through the years I had grown in my faith and understanding of God and Jesus, but I had never heard anything like what I was now hearing from this man! It was not that I did not believe him. In fact, what I was hearing, arrested my attention. It was like I was thirsting for what I was hearing but had not known it until I heard it. I just needed him to slow down some, because it was like trying to drink from a fire hose!

I left Dr. Jones and the restaurant with his jacket and a signed copy of the book *The Coming Crisis*. Good choice Dr. Jones. It was the smallest and easiest to read of all his books. I stopped everything that afternoon and night to read it through.

And so I made **two resolutions**. First, since I was on a quest for truth in every area of my life, **I needed to know more truth about my faith from this man**. And second, that God, or Yehovah as I could now call Him by name, had gifted me this opportunity to know important new things - so I would have to approach this very matter-of-factly as I wanted **no romantic involvement.**

I was doing well with my first resolution - but that second resolution did not hold up!

So here we were. We had actually planned to marry eighteen months after we first met, but just weeks before the wedding date, I got a clear red light from Yehovah to STOP! This was devastating for Miles but a huge relief to me. We broke up, but a couple of months later I agreed to get back together with him. For a whole year Miles did not bring up the subject of marriage, which I was most grateful for. Then, it seemed like he was asking me every other week! All I knew to say to him was, "*I can't marry you. Not until I get a green light from Yehovah."* This felt safe and secure for me. I was in no rush and knew I was on solid and unquestionable ground. I knew I must always listen and try not to miss anything of Father's guidance to me.

At the end of 2022, I started learning Hebrew from our Benai Emunah Hebrew teacher Jenny Webster. I had made a preliminary start with Miles by getting familiar with the Hebrew letters, sounds, various words and names, but I was a Hebrew language beginner. One of the first things Jenny taught me was the Aaronic blessing. Miles thought it was crazy to teach a beginner the Aaronic blessing. It was indeed difficult to learn and memorize. I cannot remember if this was Jenny's idea or mine, but I wanted to learn it and was absolutely committed to learning it.

Jenny was patient and persevering! Over and over and over again I would practice the sounds, the words, the phrases, the lines, then eventually the whole blessing. Why was I so desiring and committed to learning this blessing that even Miles had not learned? I even ended up teaching this blessing to him!

Initially, I did not know if it was possible that I would get to go on this archaeological survey of Mount Sinai. It was financially costly, requiring funds I did not have. My friend Janice Baca, the Translation Team Leader, felt similarly. We reassured our hearts that Father would make a way to Mount Sinai for those He wanted there. Miles however was simply confident that I would go. I was seeing the miracle of others having their costs met in incredible ways. One day Janice told me that I should just prepare as if I was going because she was certain I would be. So I did. Janice herself had prayed, "*Abba, please make a way for us to go to Mount Sinai.*" Yehovah heard her petition. On November 3rd, Janice and her husband David, were gifted with an all expenses paid trip to Mount Sinai.

Then there was Danielle's story, another friend who had learned of this upcoming expedition to Mount Sinai in the Benai Emunah newsletter. Her heart had immediately longed to go. As a young mother homeschooling their son, going on such a trip would leave no one to care for him while her husband was at work. She put her desire in Father's hands and spoke nothing of it to her husband. Several weeks later, her husband surprised her by saying, "*I saw a newsletter about a trip to Mount Sinai. I think you should go. I will look after Isaac.*" And so Danielle was to come, another miracle!

I had been sending out information of this epic adventure journey to people and answering many emails of inquiry. Not only would this be a tour, but an extension week was being offered to anyone who would like to join Dr. Jones on an Archaeological Survey of Mount Sinai and the surrounding areas in Midian.

Neither Covid jabs or Covid tests were required - an assurance we all wanted before signing up! And sign up they did. Very soon we had sufficient compensation funds for my travel costs to be met. That was a joyful day for me!

By now, we had 15 women that would be going. I suggested to Janice that we invite them to a Zoom call. Perhaps the women might even like to regularly meet together by Zoom, prior to our epic journey. It would be a great way to build relationships and know each other prior to leaving, I thought. And so we did. The *Women of Sinai* met weekly, for the two months prior. It was here we shared information and ideas on travel, clothing, climbing necessities and accessories, physical training strategies. It was here we spoke our questions, concerns and wonderings. It was here we prayed and shared Scripture together. It was here we shared how The Spirit was speaking to our hearts. It was here we shared the dreams we'd had and the visions we had seen regarding our Mount Sinai journey. And since Dr. Jones had brought to our attention that Psalm 24 actually referred to Mount Sinai, it was here in our women's weekly zoom calls that we realized Father was gathering His daughters for a special purpose on this trip. To lead in worship and purity of heart.

Psalm 24 became our focus, our meditation, our standard and our dreaming. **Psalm 24 became the central focus in our spiritual preparations.**

THE KING OF GLORY

Psalm 24 - A Psalm of David

The Earth is Yehovah's, and all its fullness,
The world and those who dwell therein.
For He has founded it upon the seas,
And established it upon the waters.
Who may ascend into the hill of Yehovah?
Or who may stand in His holy place?

He who has clean hands and a pure heart,
Who has not lifted up his soul to an idol, nor sworn deceitfully.
He shall receive blessing from Yehovah,
And righteousness from the God of his salvation.
This is Jacob, the generation of those who seek Him,
Who seek Your face. Selah

Lift up your heads, O you portals (gates)!
And be lifted up, you everlasting portals (doors)!
And the King of glory shall come in.

Who is this King of glory?
Yehovah strong and mighty,
Yehovah mighty in battle.
Lift up your heads, O you portals (gates)!
Lift up, you everlasting portals (doors)!
And the King of glory shall come in.

Who is this King of glory?
Yehovah-Tzva'ot, He is the King of glory. *Selah*

While some of the women had many dreams and visions, I had just three short dreams. On January 18th, 2023, I had a dream where these words were spoken to me in a clarion voice, "***There is more ahead of you than time would suggest Fiona.***" I am now known by my middle name Cate, but Fiona is my given name. I did not know what this could mean, and if this pertained to my immediate future or not, but I was told it was important to take notice when spoken to by name. This quickly brought to my mind the words of Scripture:

Fear not, for I have redeemed you;
I have called you by your name; You are Mine.
Isaiah 43:1

I kept this divine message from the dream in my heart, and whenever it came to mind, I tried to remember to say, "*Hineini.*"

Hineini is Hebrew and means *I am ready Yehovah. Here I am.*

On February 14, 2023, I had a second dream. **A selection of different shades of blue linens were put before me and I was to choose one. I then saw the word ISAIAH**.

Linen is Yehovah's choice fabric. He created it with extremely high frequency, and because this frequency is so much higher than that of our body, it raises our body's energy and promotes health. "*The priest shall then put on his linen clothes, with linen undergarments next to his body...*" (Leviticus 6:10)

Blue can represent Yehovah, or something dedicated to a holy purpose. It can also symbolize royalty or riches. We see this most in the book of Exodus (34 times). *Blue* can also mean or symbolize service to God and Godly living. *Holiness.* I did not know how Isaiah might relate, as I could not find a scriptural link between ***blue, linen*** and ***Isaiah,*** but this verse from Isaiah 35:8 came to mind - "*A highway shall be there and a road, and it shall be called the Highway of Holiness. The unclean shall not pass over it, but it shall be for others.*"

During Janice's prayer time one morning in the middle of February, she saw a vision of Esther coming before the king. Why was she given this vision? Then she realized – Purim was approaching. Janice wondered if it would be around the time we were going to Mount Sinai. She was shocked to discover that not only would it be taking place at the time of our trip, but we were scheduled to climb Mount Sinai on the third day of Purim. So, we would be presenting ourselves to the King of the Universe on the same day that Esther presented herself to her king!

Janice called me to share the exciting news. I said, "*Janice, what is the Torah portion for that **week**?*"

[The Torah, also known as the Five Books of Moses or the Pentateuch, is divided into 54 separate portions and linked to a specific week of the year. From the time of Ezra till today, these weekly portions are read aloud in synagogues and Messianic assemblies on Shabbat and speak prophetically even into our modern times.]

She responded, "*Cate, what is the Torah portion for that* ***day****?*" Incredibly, the Torah portion during our visit to Mount Sinai was Exodus 33:17-23 - the passage describing Moses hiding in the cleft of the rock to see the glory of Yehovah pass before him!

But He said, "You cannot see My face;
for no man shall see Me, and live...
Here is a place by Me, and you shall stand on the rock.
So it shall be, while My glory passes by,
that I will put you in the cleft of the rock,
and will cover you with My hand while I pass by."
Exodus 33:20-22

Yehovah passed by, Moses saw His glory, granting his request! We wondered if this was a sign that miracles would happen when we, too, came to Mount Sinai?

As Janice shared her excitement with the group, others decided to join us in fasting and prayer even as Esther's people had joined her. We were preparing to go before Yehovah at Mount Sinai. As Psalm 24 said, only those with clean hands and a pure heart could ascend Har Yehovah. And so we prepared with prayer.

Prayer was not our only preparation. And while this tour was being organized by a travel company, there was also a lot of individual and group planning, organizing and preparation for the journey.

We needed suitable cotton / linen clothing, as well as gloves, hats, shoes, head coverings for the women, First Aid and medicinal items, travel toilet paper and hand sanitizer. To climb Mount Sinai required boots, pants, hiking sticks, day packs, camelback water bags for hydration, electrolytes, and energy snacks. Then there were all things electronic: phones, cameras, chargers, memory cards, adapters, as well as filming and audio equipment, for filming and photographing. And finally, we needed inscription charts, reference material, pens, markers, small plastic bags for collection of findings, and a whole host of miscellaneous items.

We had Zoom meetings to give information and training to those team members staying on for the week of research in and around Mount Sinai. If we did not already know, we were to learn Google Earth and how to follow a pin or lay a pin during our journey. A pin is a location that someone has identified as being important. We would otherwise have no idea what we were walking over as we walked through the archeological areas. We would be documenting the co-ordinates of previously found inscriptions, as well as surveying the areas where we would look for inscriptions of the Israelites. We wanted everyone to be as involved as much as they wanted to be.

There was organizing and booking of flights to and from Washington DC, as well as required accommodation while still in the USA. Passports and other required travel documentation were obtained. We needed to organize international calling on cell phones, and for some of us women, we learned to play and practiced our kalimbas - small thumb pianos for worship of Yehovah together.

Important too, was to familiarize ourselves with the rules and etiquette we would need to follow in Saudi Arabia. For example, men were not to engage in a conversation with a Saudi woman. Women were to dress modestly with loose-fitted clothing - knees, shoulders or décolleté were not to be exposed. We were not to eat, pass, or receive food with our left hand. We were not to show the bottom of our feet (with shoes or without) as it is considered rude to sit with your leg up and crossed with the bottom of your feet showing. We were also to be aware that Saudi Arabia had no private or public religious freedom for non-Muslims, and this included us.

So it was a big job to plan, purchase and pack everything Miles and I would both need. Exciting and fun too! We would be there in spring, and temperatures would fluctuate from mid-80's°F during the day to low 30's at night.

The item I most wanted to take was my ram's horn, or *Yovel*. It is after all, what evokes the power and blessing of Yehovah when it is sounded. Yet we were told we could not bring any shofars as they would be confiscated by Saudi authorities on entry into the country, or worse still, jeopardize our team being allowed entry into Saudi Arabia. While disappointed by this restriction, we comforted ourselves knowing there was a *Yovel* hidden somewhere on Mount Sinai for us to find. And find it we would!

As Janice prepared for Mount Sinai, her friend asked that a white handkerchief be placed upon the Mountain of God for the healing of her blind eyes, and this idea went viral! Between the group members, we brought about 200 handkerchiefs to touch the altar of Yehovah on Sinai! Names were either written, embroidered, or left blank for all who would receive a handkerchief. Janice spent weeks embroidering names on each handkerchief. For the extra handkerchiefs, she embroidered the name of Yehovah!

As our departure date approached, excitement grew and spread throughout our Benai Emunah Institute volunteers and the Mount Sinai group. Congruently with these preparations, another team at Benai Emunah was formed, led by John Reed-Austin. Their focus was to restore the original biblical songs - the Mizmorim. Their first song would be Psalm 24. A global choir of volunteers was quickly brought together by Jonathan Felt, who added their voices to the recording of Psalm 24 completed by the Mizmorim team. This was to be played at Mount Sinai.

On February 27, 2023, just three days before Miles and I were to leave, my friend Renae came to visit. Renae is an anointed daughter of The Most High who shakes the spiritual darkness when she prays and worships. Her love for Israel and the Jewish people is great, and she has made dozens of visits to Israel. Knowing of Miles' and my imminent journey to Mount Sinai, she had driven from her nearby town to make an unexpected special delivery. I was looking forward to sharing my excitement of the wonderful Yehovah-happenings related to this trip, and to have her pray with me for all matters pertaining to this very strenuous time of preparation. She knew it was taking a heavy toll on me, in spite of how wonderful it all was.

Time spent with Renae was always a blessing, but today's visit would bring me special encouragement and joy. She told me she had some special things to loan me for this trip. She then proceeded to take two big silk worship flags out of a bag. Both were gorgeous and amazing, but especially the one that had Yeshua's name across it. Then Renae paused momentarily and said in a more intimate, almost sacred tone, "*the other thing I have for you to borrow is something I have never released to anyone else, but God has told me that He wants you to take this to Mount Sinai.*" Renae carefully took something out of the bag as she said, "*This is my Queen Esther belt. There is a special purpose for you with this. I don't know what it is, but you will find out.*"

Wait, what?... did she just say, "*Queen Esther*"? As in... the **'Queen Esther of Purim'?**

This was to be the latest piece of *'incredible'* regarding this journey. I'd had no previous conversation with Renae about Janice's Purim dream. And Renae was not aware that we would be at Mount Sinai for Purim! I knew this was going to be good!

I had not heard of an Esther belt before. I was most eager to know more. Renae began to tell that it was a holy garment and that until now, she had not loaned it to anyone. She told me that Yehovah Himself released the belt to me. She put the belt on me. It was very beautiful... A soft wine-colored sash with small gold bells either end. She had wrapped the fabric twice around my waist. The bell ends hung low on the side of my body. With even just a little movement of my body, the bell's delicate sound could be heard. It was very beautiful!

"*It's worn to bring the essence of Yehovah's presence where He desires dominion,*" Renae told me. "*It's a tangible visual, that changes the atmosphere through His Presence and His Directives.*" She added a caution, that Yehovah demands obedience, and the belt was only to be worn when He directs, and for His purposes.

Of course I was riveted, as Renae told me the incredible story of this beautiful belt - how she had been guided step by step through the Old City of Jerusalem to a certain merchant where she got it. Each time she had worn it, highly significant - even miraculous - experiences had come with it. With Renae, this did not surprise me at all. Still, I was gob smacked.

When I eventually got to tell Renae of Janice's Purim dream, and that we were actually going to be camped at our King's Mountain on Purim, her eyes twinkled as she smiled and said, "*Well... what more confirmation do you need!*"

Renae told me her prayers were that I would have the adventure of a lifetime. She told me that worship was key. She told me that Yehovah would guide me and keep me every step of the way. She told me that I did not have to be concerned about my physical limitations and that all I needed to do was to "show up." Before she left my home, Renae prayed over me and blessed me. I would not see Renae again until we got back from Mount Sinai.

On the 4th of March 2023 Miles and I flew from San Antonio to Washington D.C. We would be there four days before the rest of our team arrived. This provided opportunity for Miles to research, and for us to meet with the Curator of the 'Museum Of The Bible.' Alice was one of the women traveling to Saudia Arabia with us. She lived in Washington D.C. near the Dulles International Airport, where we would be leaving from. Her kindness to host Miles and I was a huge blessing and help, as we would require two rooms.

The day before our departure, Alice rang me to check that I had my USA Residency Card, knowing that I'd need it to return to the USA. Oh no… I could not believe that I had left it at home in Texas! I rang our tour company operator and explained the situation. Her response was clear. She told me I should not go on the trip but return home instead. She knew from previous experience that without my Residency Card I would not be allowed back into the USA when we returned. She told me nothing was worth that situation happening. I did not like that advice at all - what a huge blow!

At the time, Miles and I were at the Library of Congress, and Miles was in deep discussion with Dr. Yohannes Zeleke, who would also be on our trip. On this matter I was not reluctant to interrupt. The alarm in my voice was more than an acceptable library whisper and we were directed by the librarian to take our conversation out into the corridor. Here, I informed Miles that I did not have my Residency Card, and that Rhonda had determined I should not pursue this trip. Instead to go home. Miles immediately declared, *"That's not happening. I need you with me. You're going!"*

So I called Janice and David. They lived 40 minutes from my house. I fully expected them to have already departed for D.C. Instead, they were loaded up in their truck and about to leave for the airport. I told Janice the situation and Rhonda's advice to me. Janice didn't miss a beat and was just as adamant as Miles. She declared, "*Well that sure isn't happening! Yehovah has purposed you to be at His mountain, and you WILL be there!*"

They immediately drove to our town of Kerrville where I lived, and to my house where my neighbor happened to be home - and she had my house key. Janice was able to enter my house and locate my Residency Card. Then she and David still got to the airport in San Antonio in time for their flight to DC from where we were all departing to Saudi Arabia. Praise Yehovah!

The precise timing of all this happening was something to consider. If I had called even a few minutes later, they would have already left their rural property and headed out in a completely different direction. They may not have had cell phone service to even get my call! And should I have simply given into the idea that I should not go to Saudi because of me being refused entry back into the USA at the border, this would have meant forfeiting the place where Father wanted me to be. Where He had very special plans for me.

Together with our film crew, some of our Benai Emunah team, and many new friends, we had a total of 35 people embarking on an adventure that would result in miracles at Mount Sinai. Miracles we could never have imagined that Yehovah had purposed.

The 12-hour flight from Washington D.C. to Jeddah, Saudi Arabia, was arduous, so it was a great relief to land. We then took a connecting flight to the small airport of Tabuk where our Land Cruiser drivers were waiting for us. This was March 6, 2023.

After stopping at a restaurant for a delicious Saudi smorgasbord, we were taken to the brand-new Millennium Hotel. We were all super tired and it was after midnight before we got to bed. With only a few hours of sleep, Miles arose for a 6:00 am meeting with a Saudi gentleman. The meeting would prove to be mind-blowing. As Miles related to me, "*After introductions, the man immediately reached into his bag and pulled out an ancient book with paleo-Hebrew writing embossed on pages of beaten gold! The first thing I saw was a large circular seal on the cover of the gold book with the Name of YHVH written in the ancient alphabet! That was better than a cup of coffee to wake me up!*" There were many other books written on lead tablets. These were the archives of the Bene Quareza, a Hebrew priestly tribe fleeing Roman persecution from Israel to Mecca in the second century AD.

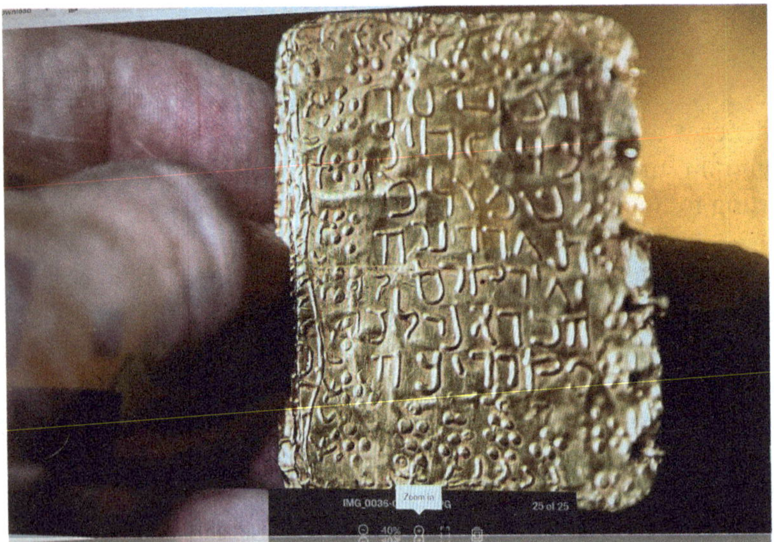

The beaten gold book with paleo-Hebrew writing

2025 Spiritual Awakening: As I was rereading this chapter prior to publication, The Spirit of Yehovah brought this Scripture to my mind. Abba's loving-kindness to show this to me, has *deeply* moved me:

But He knows the way that I take;
***When** He has tested me, I shall come forth as gold.*
Job 23:10

I too am now ***beaten gold,*** with His WORD - **His Torah** - His signet, **written on my heart!** (see Jeremiah 31:33)
My Creator **holds *me* in *HIS HAND*** and **I am a treasure to Him.**

*****

And so here we were in Saudi Arabia where the foundational narrative of the Exodus, as outlined in the book of Exodus, contained some of the most vital and epoch-making accounts in all the Tanakh (Old Testament). Our objective was to find the archaeological and geological evidence of the Israelites' deliverance from Egypt, Moses' revelation at Mount Sinai, and the nation of Israel's ensuing desert wanderings. Later, we came to learn that these very stories were related in the Gold Book of the Bene Quareza in the ancient alphabet of the Israelites, on the FIRST DAY of our expedition to Sinai!

Land of Midian, Saudi Arabia

In the first week of time in Saudi Arabia, we explored the Land of Hagar, Jethro and Moses. We went to Jethro's Caves and the well of Moses and Zipporah. We examined and hiked up the majestic Split Rock of Horeb at Jabal Maqla. Here, Moses struck the boulder and Yehovah miraculously provided water from within. It was breathtaking to see! We went to the peak of Jabal Maqla, Moses' Altar, where the pillar stones representing the 12 tribes of Israel are found, and to Aaron's Golden Calf Altar. We explored the cemetery that is dated back to the time of the Exodus and saw the standing stones of ancient times that mark the grave sites. We drove through the Land of the Amalekites. We reached Elim – the place of 12 wells and 70 palms - by an off-road visit through the meandering open valleys most likely tread by the Israelites. Some of us had the incredible experience of walking from Elim through the Wadi al Tayyib to the Red Sea gateway. We also saw the beach directly across from Nuweiba.

This meant some long hours spent in our Land Cruisers each day, but everything to me was captivating in the dark red windswept landscape. And throughout our time in Saudi Arabia, the NEOM project was in full swing. NEOM is the ultra-modern city they are building right beside Mount Sinai.

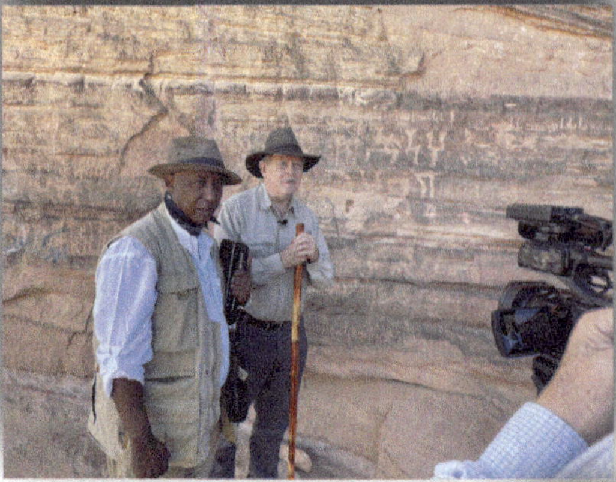

Filming at
Jethro's Caves
with Dr. Jones & Dr. Zeleke

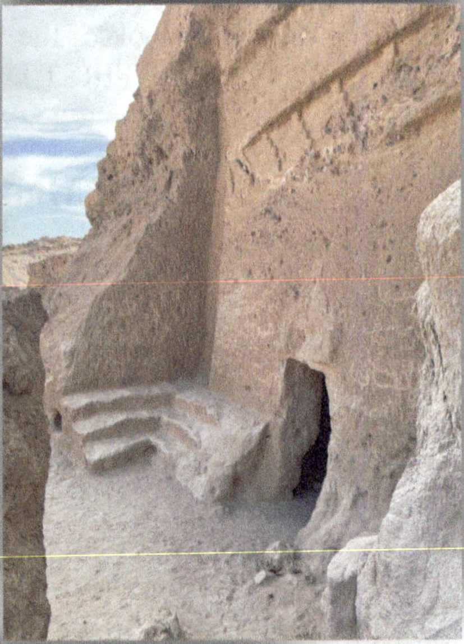

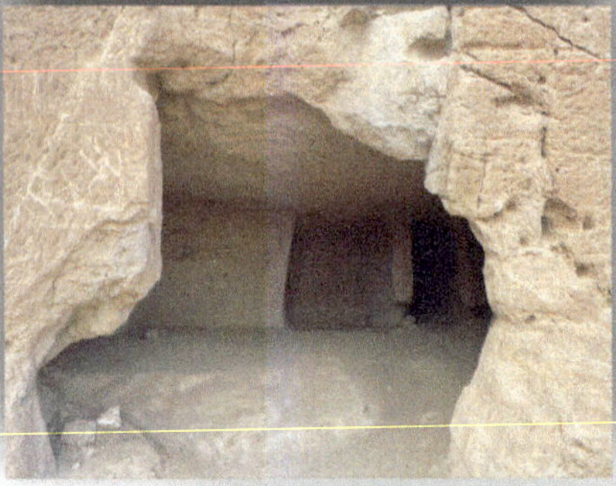

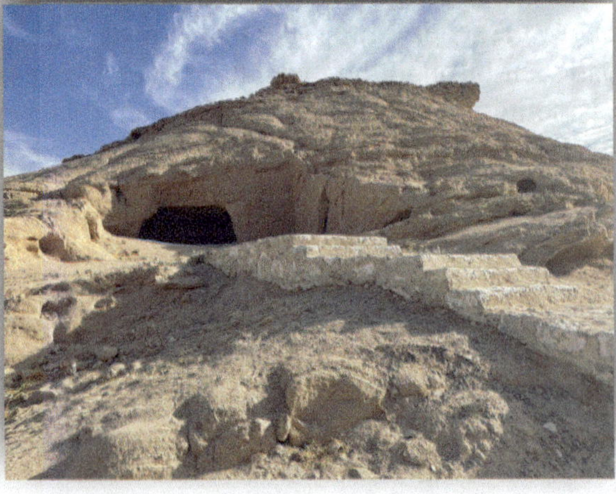

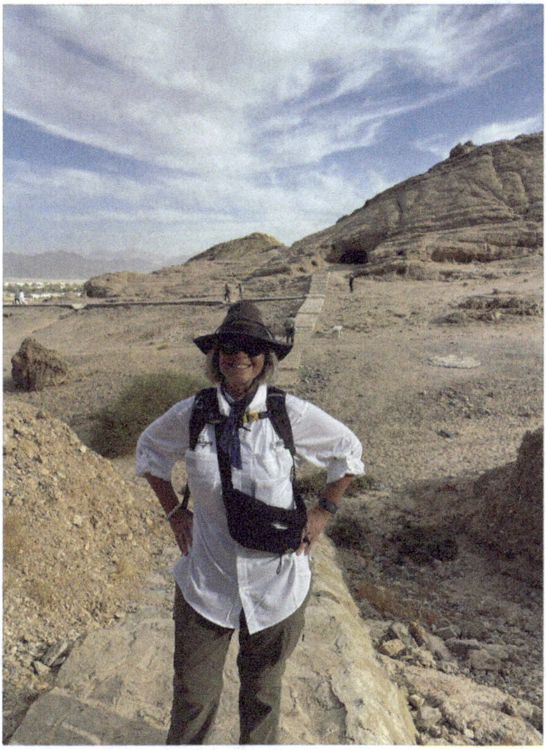

Cate at Jethro's Caves
Dr. Jones at the Majestic Split Rock of Horeb at Jabal Maqla

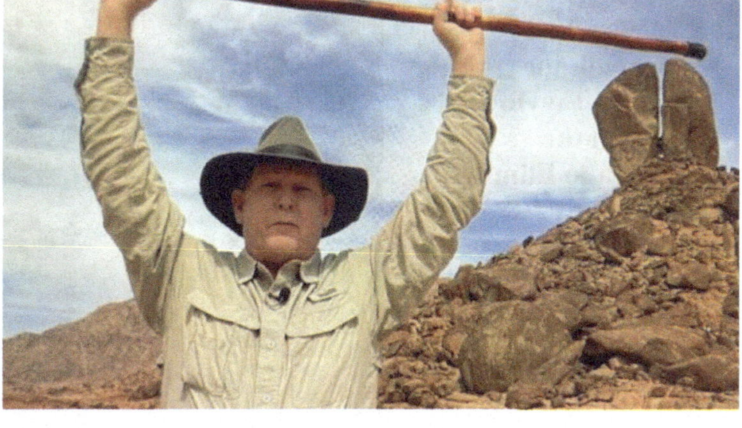

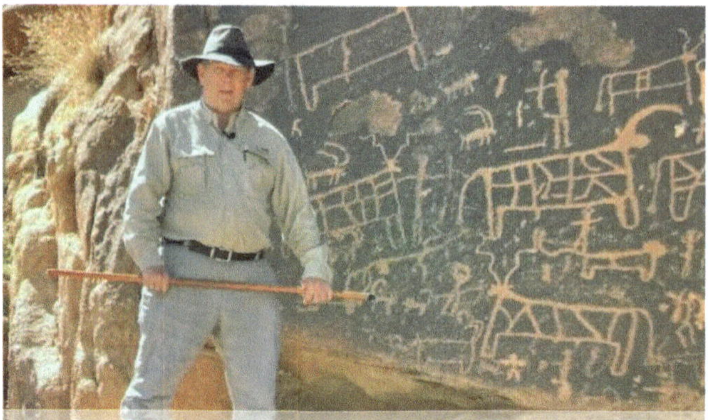

Above:
Dr. Jones
Filming Inscriptions

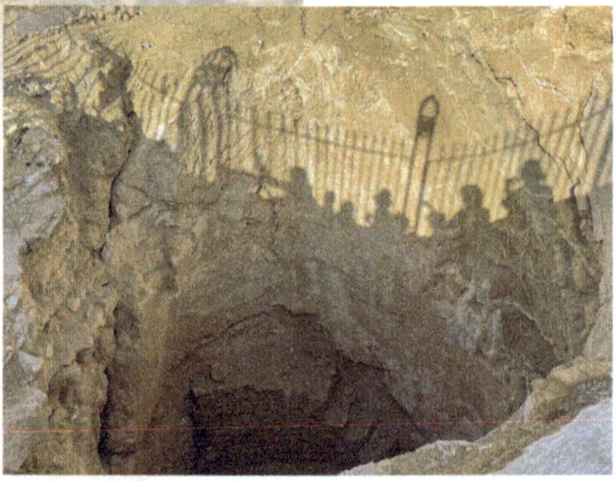

Middle:
Moses & Zipporah's
well

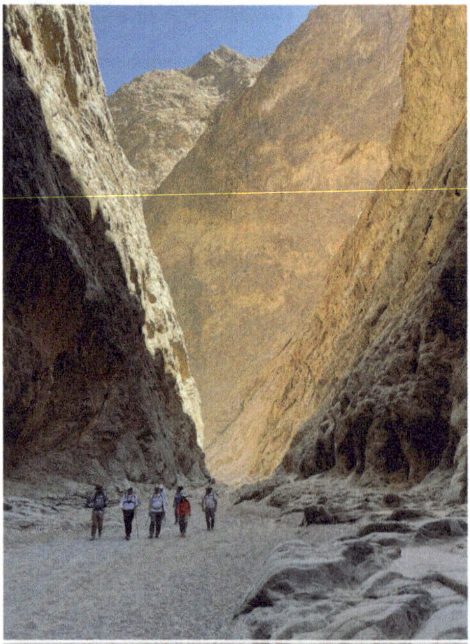

Right:
We walked
through the
Wadi al Tayyib
from the
Red Sea to Elim

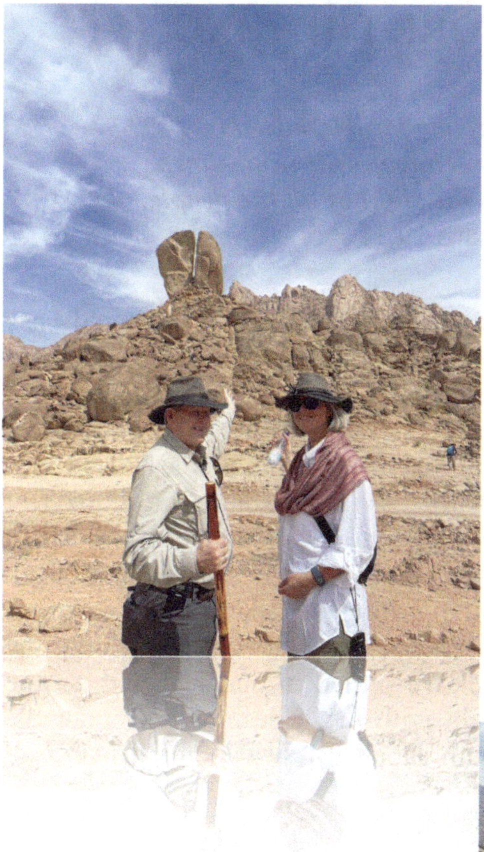

The Majestic Split Rock of Horeb

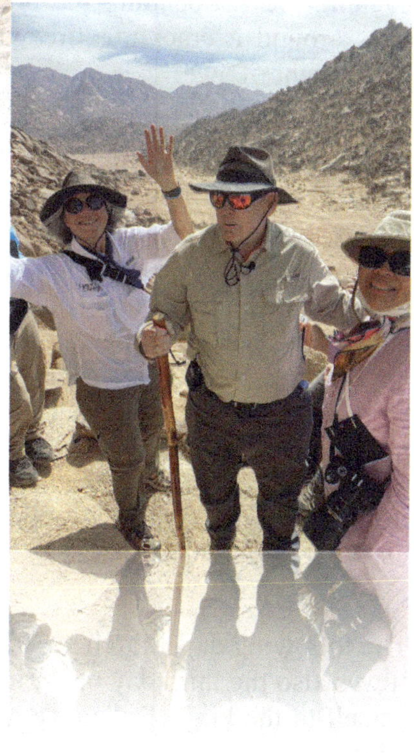

Climbing to where Moses struck the rock and water gushed out

GOING BEFORE THE KING

And let them be ready for the third day.
For on the third day ***Yehovah will come down***
upon Mount Sinai in the sight of all the people*.*
Exodus 19:11

On March 8, 2023 we went off-road to the specially prepared base camp at the foot of Mount Sinai, Jabal al-Lawz (meaning the almond mountain in Arabic) for the night. Jabal al-Lawz is hailed as one of the most mysterious mountains in the Middle East (with Maqla its highest peak). Most people think that Saudi Arabia is a land of vast sand dunes, but this is far from true. With its summit at 8,362 feet above sea level, Jabal al- Lawz is the highest mountain of the Tabuk Province. Jabal al-Lawz is now known to be the real Mount Sinai. This is where Moses received the writing of God and the covenant commandments, meeting Him in a cloud of fire scorching the mountaintop. And here we were! We settled in our tents and ate the evening meal. Spending the night with the tribesmen out under the stars around a crackling fire with Jabal al-Lawz looming overhead was a sight of awe.

The Saudis had set up a karaoke speaker expecting to play Saudi secular music through the evening. However, our group had a different idea. We gathered singers, dancers, Bluetooth speakers, tambourines, thumb pianos and raced outside the camp to worship Yehovah! With surround-sound speakers at the entrance of our tent compound, we worshipped, danced, and sang Mizmor 24, also lifting up our hearts and voices in prayer. Not one person stopped our worship and prayer for the 90 minutes we were there! And what's more, Yehovah graced us with an enormous full moon over the mountain that night that bathed us all in moonlight! And it was here that I had put on the Esther belt. I believed this was ***the*** occasion I was purposed to wear the belt!

The following day, March 9, 2023, was **our first day at Mount Sinai**. It was also the third day of Purim. The same day that Esther presented herself to the king! Today, we were going to present ourselves to The King!

It was our greatly anticipated climbing the mountain day! And it was climbing, not hiking. We were to be physically fit. The climb was advanced. So in the months prior, those intending to make the ascent had been in physical training. The Plateau of the 70 Elders would take around 6-7 hours round-trip, Elijah's Cave 7-8 hours round-trip, and the Blackened Peak 7-8 hours round-trip. It wasn't possible to get to both the peak and Elijah's Cave, so we had to chose whether we climb to Elijah's cave, the Plateau of the Elders, or to the Peak of Mount Sinai. My desire and determination for the past months had been to reach the Plateau of the Elders, and I had done my best to be ready for this.

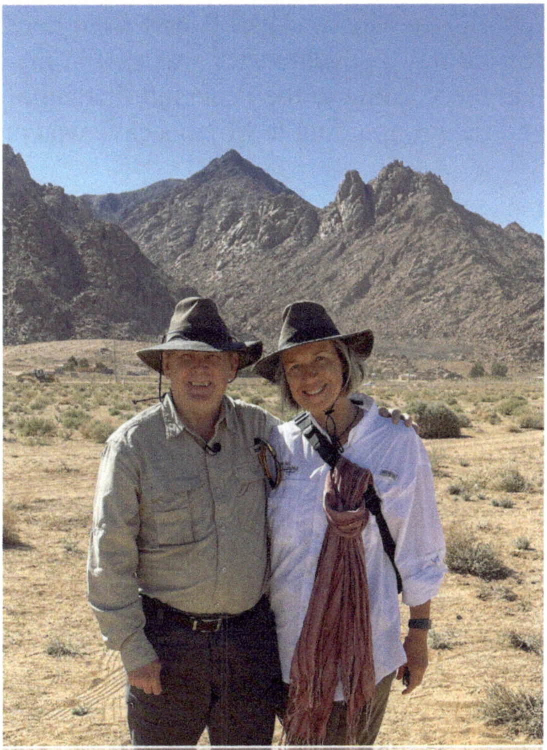

Standing in front of Mount Sinai, Jabal al-Lawz

After breakfast we all gathered for instructions and the pep talk on climbing the mountain. It had been an extremely cold night in our tents, but now the sun and risen and there was not a cloud in the sky. It appeared to be the most perfect day to climb Har Yehovah! Necessary but deflating was the very stern advice given by Rhonda our tour leader, that no one should attempt to climb the mountain if they had any doubt whatsoever about out their capability or wellness. She reminded us that recently even some accomplished climbers had got into trouble on the mountain and had either jeopardized the safety of their co-climbers or it had meant the whole team had to forfeit going further. Someone had even required an air lift off the mountain.

So while I laced up my boots, put on my camel-back pack with ample water, grabbed my climbing gloves, hat and wet neck tie, I was completely uncertain about my ability to ascend Yah's mountain after setting my heart on this for many months! I knew that those who didn't climb would have plenty to explore on flatter ground and small mounds that mysteriously could hide secrets of the past. Miles was not climbing, he was filming, so I considered not climbing too.

Our team drove to the base of Mount Sinai so we could then walk the foothills to Moses' Altar. It was from here that we would all separate for our day's adventures. I was still in my indecision, when I realized that those going to the Peak and Plateau of the elders had already left, and the group going to Elijah's cave was just heading off.

I found myself hurriedly saying goodbye to Miles before running to catch up and get in step with Roland and Lilian Atencio, and the four young Saudi men who would be our guides up the rugged mountain to Elijah's cave.

There is only one cave on the mountain that is very noticeable from the ground level. It is seen on the front of the mountain, above the altar of Moses and the 12 pillars. According to 1 Kings chapter 19, the prophet Elijah stayed in a cave on Mount Sinai and interacted with Yehovah there. He was fleeing Ahab and Jezebel in fear of his life.

Elijah had traveled 40 days and 40 nights to Mount Sinai, and once there, he found a cave to sleep in that night. The next day, Yehovah instructed Elijah to "*go out and stand on the mountain in the presence of Adonai, for Adonai is about to pass by.*"

A great wind then caused falling rocks, an earthquake, and a fire. Elijah, however, was protected as Adonai was not "*in*" the phenomenon. Once the dangerous weather subsided, Elijah heard a "*gentle whisper*" from Yehovah and "*pulled a cloak over his face and went out and stood at the mouth of the cave.*"

Immediately I knew this climb would be challenging even with two climbing poles. The whole mountain was rocks and loose stones, and it was steep! There was no trail. But… I was ascending the mountain of Har Yehovah! How surreal. I was living Psalm 24! What a privilege, joy and blessing. It had been my heart's desire to do this, and now I was!

We were very pleased and grateful to have the help of our four Saudi guides who were there to get us safely up and down the mountain. They appeared to know very little English, yet that didn't seem to be a problem. They were friendly and responsive to our communication efforts.

Once the climbers had set off, Dr. Jones finished a video recording at the altar, and some of our women team members placed dozens of white handkerchiefs on and among the rocks of Moses' Altar. They praised Yehovah and prayed over these small tokens – asking for miracles like those that followed Paul. Janice of course, was one of the women.

Now God worked unusual miracles by the hands of Paul,
so that even ***handkerchiefs*** *or aprons*
were brought from his body to the sick,
and the diseases left them and the evil spirits went out of them.
Acts 19:11-12

Actually, they had surround-sound speakers at the altar and worshipped, danced, and sang – loudly and boldly! Not once did they look over their shoulders in fear. In fact, our American tour guide said she looked for the Saudis and realized they were nowhere to be found!

The climb was indeed challenging. It took us 7-8 hours. There were no trails to follow, we were making a steep ascent on loose stones and rocks. Each of our groups did so with the experience of at least several Saudi men as guides, and we relied on them to scout out the best and safest way up and down the mountain.

Halfway up to Elijah's cave, I realized something was seriously wrong! While I was not out of breath from exertion, and my legs were doing just fine - my heart started to go berserk! With the first sense of it, I slowed down. Then very quickly my heart was experiencing a full attack. I was now at the back of our small group, and with some distance between me and others. One of the guides was with me. The crushing pressure on my heart was severe. I immediately stopped. All I could do was pant with short shallow breaths in an attempt to calm the berserk-ness going on in my heart and relieve the crushing sensation. What was happening? Is this a heart attack!

The guide who was with me didn't appear to speak English. He seemed to assume I was only tired and just needed to catch my breath. Yet the one thing he did know to say in English was, *"Take your time, take your time."* I could only very quietly say, "*It's my heart,*" but he did not understand and repeated with a smile, "*Take your time, take your time.*" After a few minutes my heart settled somewhat, so I very slowly started to climb again. But after three more big steps up on the rocks that required all my effort, even with the help of climbing poles, my heart was again in great pain and going berserk. Was this because of the myocarditis I'd had some years back that had left my heart muscle scarred?

I had not even given this heart history a single thought during the whole time of preparing for Mount Sinai and the climb. Even while on the mountain and experiencing this distress, I did not put two and two together. It would only be once I was back in the USA, that I would learn that high altitude can be dangerous - even fatal - for someone with residual heart scarring from myocarditis. This is because the heart's function is already compromised, and high altitudes further strain the heart.

Lilian, Roland and the other guides were just far enough ahead that I couldn't explain was happening. They also thought I was just tired and needed to rest, so they weren't concerned but focused on their challenge of climbing. I remember the thoughts and conversations with Yehovah I had while this was happening…

"I think I could die on Your mountain!"

"What an incredible place to die!"

"Yehovah, if I die here that's absolutely fine with me."

"If You want me at Elijah's cave, You will need to get me there."

And so, from halfway up the mountain until I reached the cave with my guide, I contended with my heart going beserk and having to stop every two or three steep steps up. And still none of the group knew what was happening to me, and still my guide repeated over and over "*Take your time. Take your time.*"

As I saw the cave getting closer, my mind was focused on praising and thanking Yehovah. He was indeed *giving His angels charge over me to keep me in all my ways* (Psalm 91:11-12). I was getting there.

Once I got to the entrance of the cave my heart was immediately well. Any thoughts of me, were replaced by the sheer thrill of where I was! I was now below the cleft of the rock where Yehovah put Moses and covered him while His glory passed by (Exodus 33: 21-23). And I was now at the entrance of the cave where Elijah had come and received Yehovah's revelation. The cave where Moses and Abraham may also have been! Perhaps Paul too. THEY had all climbed this holy mountain of Yehovah and possibly come here to this cave for refuge… And now I had too. **H.o.w I.n.c.r.e.d.i.b.l.e!**

Looking out from Elijah's Cave

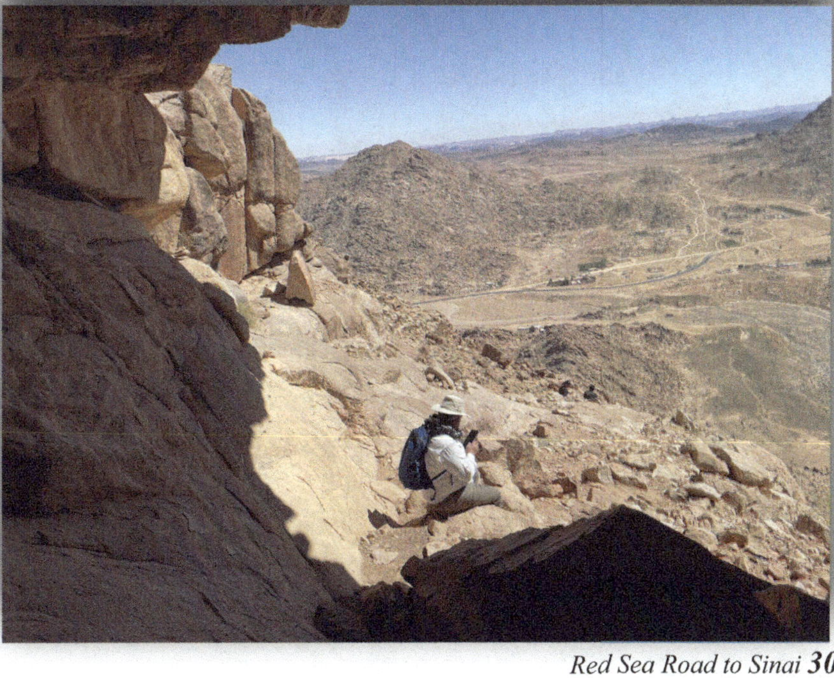

So few people in the world, so few children of Israel throughout all the centuries, have *ever* climbed this holy mountain or been in this cave. Yet multitudes of people have read many times over about Elijah's cave, only to imagine what it would be like! **How was it possible that I was here?**

Giddy with joy and wonder, I slowly moved into the cave. It was the size of a small bedroom - about 15 feet high, 20 feet wide and 20 feet deep. The top of the cave decreased from 15 feet to about 8 feet as I went further into the back of the cave. I imagined myself sleeping here. It would definitely be safe and comfortable!

While I might have had my feet on different rocks and stones as I climbed the mountain to get here, now in the cave I was definitely placing my hands and feet where Elijah and Moses would have stood, sat, slept, touched, prayed, ate, wept… These great men of faith… So many people I knew who would want to be **right.where.I.am.now**!

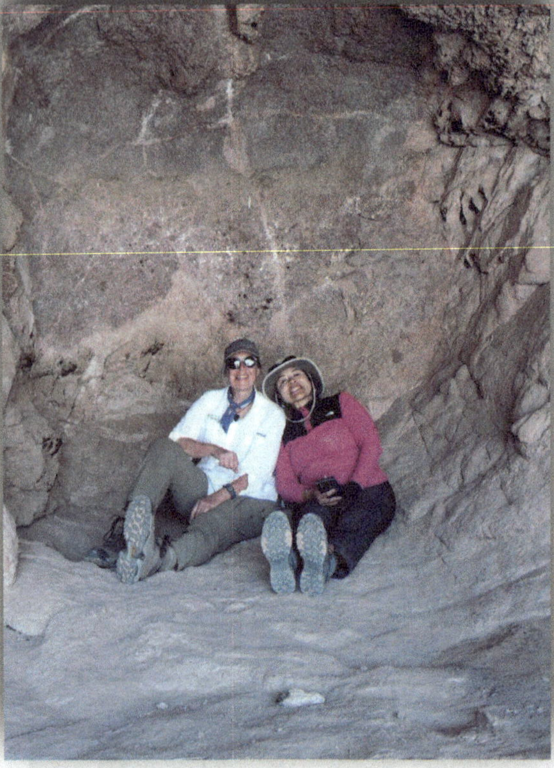

Lilian and I in the back of Elijah's Cave

Elijah had surely been tired from ascending the mountain to this cave. I too was now tired and needed rest, food and water. Here now on March 9, 2023, I, Fiona Cate 'Smith', was finding refuge in Elijah's cave.

Looking out from the mountain I had another view of the standing stones of the ancient cemetery – dated to Moses' time. I got out my phone to take photos and to video the cave and out across the great vista. It was awe inspiring. For most people, I imagine it would be a terrifying experience to be amongst falling rocks up here, as Elijah was!

Our Saudi guides gave us time. They understood that this was a deeply spiritual experience for us, as this place was significant to them too. Jewish and Bedouin traditions have continued for centuries to call this peak "The Mountain of Moses." Roland, Lilian and I ate and drank in Elijah's cave. We were quiet, prayerful, reflective, blessed.

Before we started our decent, I remembered my two dozen handkerchiefs that I had brought up to the cave with me. I gathered some sand and stones and placed them in the plastic bag with the anointed handkerchiefs. These I would later give to my friends and family. Then I stood at the opening of the cave and loudly declared the name of Yehovah. Following this, I felt moved to declare the Aaronic blessing in Hebrew out over the vista before me.

יְבָרֶכְךָ יְהֹוָה וְיִשְׁמְרֶךָ׃

Y'varekhekha Yehovah v'yishmerekha

Yehovah bless you, and keep you;

יָאֵר יְהֹוָה ׀ פָּנָיו אֵלֶיךָ וִיחֻנֶּךָּ׃

Ya'er Yehovah panav eleikha vichunekha

Yehovah make His face shine upon you,
and be gracious unto you;

יִשָּׂא יְהֹוָה ׀ פָּנָיו אֵלֶיךָ וְיָשֵׂם לְךָ שָׁלוֹם׃

Yissa Yehovah panav eleikha v'yasem l'kha shalom

Yehovah lift up His countenance upon you,
and give you shalom.

Numbers 6:24-26

What an honor, privilege and joy to declare this from His holy mountain in His language after long weeks of learning what had been so difficult for me. And I said every word without faltering! It had not at all been in my mind to do this. Later I would find out that one of our team members who ascended the mountain to the Plateau was also moved to declare the name of Yehovah and to speak out the Aaronic blessing in Hebrew, as well as one of our team members who ascended the mountain to the Peak. All three of us had been moved to do exactly the same thing!

So in all three places on the mountain that day, the Aaronic blessing was declared in the very same language with which Yehovah first gave this prayer of blessing, to Aaron for His people. And in all three places - the Plateau, at the Peak and in Elijah's cave - His name was proclaimed! Just to think…this was probably the first time Yehovah's name has been shouted from Mount Sinai in 3500 years!

What's more, there was a ram's horn (shofar) safely hidden in the rocks on Mount Sinai's peak. It had been left there by Keith Johnson who had shared with us the co-ordinates. Once found, the blast of the ram's horn was heard all the way to Moses' Altar! This sound was thrilling, but this sound was also significant! Why?

Blowing of the ram's horn, or *the Yovel* as it is called in Hebrew, is an ancient ordinance given to Israel at Mount Sinai, and the law that ordained the observance of what would be called *the Yovel* in Hebrew. The ram's horn is an instrument to mark the changing of times, the beginning and ends of eras.

In Exodus 19 there are two different horns blown at Mount Sinai. In verse 13, there is the description of the *Yovel* (יֹבֵל). Yet, in verse 19, there is the shofar (שׁוֹפָר) blast. Why the Y*ovel*? Because the Y*ovel* is the ram's horn blast of the *Jubilee*, and the word *Jubilee* comes from the Hebrew word *Yovel* ! *Jubilee* is the symbol of Yehovah's people being set free from slavery! The sounding of the shofar or ram's horn would signify the end of the forty-ninth year and bring in the fiftieth i.e. the *Yovel* or *Jubilee*. The sound of the ram's horn evokes Yehovah's power and blessings.

No one should touch them.
They must be stoned or shot with arrows.
No matter whether it's an animal or a person, it must not live.
The people may go up the mountain
only when the ram's horn (yovel) sounds a long blast.
Exodus 19:13, NOG

When the women who had remained at Moses' Altar heard the sound of the shofar, they experienced the joy of The Spirit bubbled up within them and they also boldly shouted the name of Yehovah three times!

All those within range, heard the shofar sound out over Har Yehovah for perhaps the first time in thousands of years. What an extraordinary experience this was for us all, no matter where on the mountain we were! And I believe in the spiritual realm too. I imagine that all the Heavenly beings and the great cloud of witnesses were tuned in to the sound! And who was it from our team that found and blew the Yovel? Who would be the one divinely designated to do this? It was Danielle, whose husband was at home looking after their son.

And so it was time for Lilian, Roland and I to descend the mountain from Elijah's cave with our Saudi guides. It was hard to leave. I was reluctant and sad to descend. I did not want to. I felt safe on the mountain in the embrace of my Creator. To be in Elijah's cave was a sanctuary for my soul. I tried to hold on to that feeling of wonder, strength and security.

About a third of the way down, I slipped on loose stones and fell head over heels down the mountain. I sprained my wrist. I broke my pole. I gashed my shin. I could only use one arm to finish the difficult descent. I clung to my Saudi guide Def. My other arm was in a makeshift sling. Def was a Godsend in getting me down safely.

*****

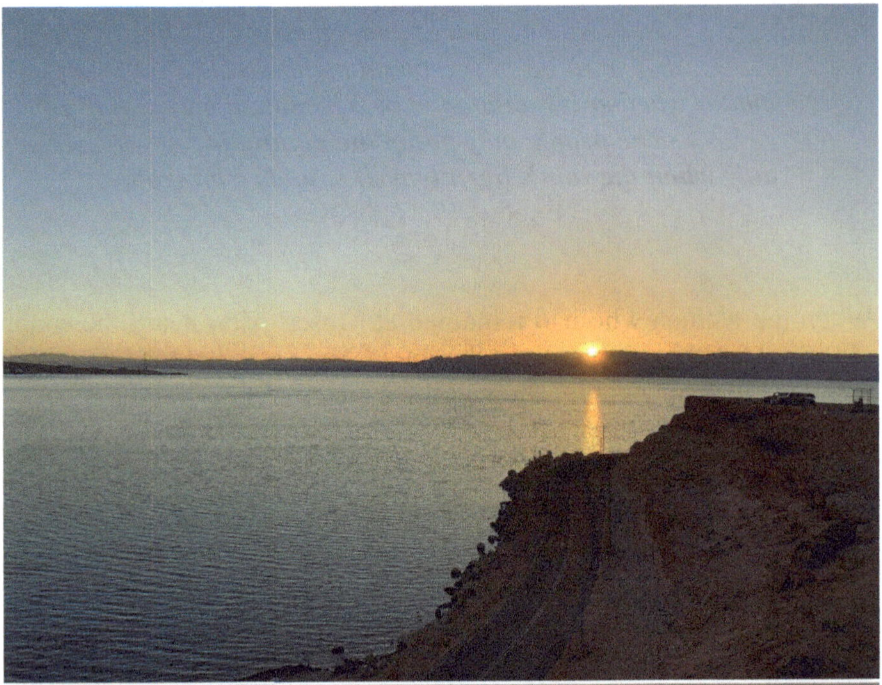

The Red Sea - view from my hotel room window

Our epic journey continued, bringing us to the Yom Suph, actually the Gulf of Aqaba - an arm of the Red Sea - in Haql.

The view of the Red Sea from my third-floor hotel room was as beautiful as it was glorious! This was the water that had been supernaturally split apart to make a path for the Israelites to escape from Pharaoh and his army. Yehovah had done this, *with a strong hand and an outstretched arm, for His mercy endures forever* (Psalm 136:12). The mighty and monumental walls of water, held back for the sake of Yehovah's beloved, were now a visual testimony to me of Yah's faithfulness to deliver. Not just having delivered the Israelites from Pharaoh, but over and over again in my life He had been my great Deliverer too. Now these waters were still, restful and shimmering in the sunshine.

On the morning of March 12, 2023, in that hotel in Haql by the Red Sea, I had a lucid dream where my spirit had an encounter with Yehovah.

I was asked, ***"Will you marry Miles?"***

I answered, ***"I can't. Things aren't ready."***

Again, I was asked, ***"Will you marry Miles?"***

Again, I responded, ***"I can't. Things aren't ready."***

A third time I was spoken to. This time I was asked, ***"Will you trust Me?"***

I answered, ***"Yes."***

It was 5:00 am when Miles knocked on my hotel room door. I was staying on the third floor and Miles was in a room on the first floor. He had heard me call his name and this awakened him from a sound sleep. Miles knew it was something supernatural, as there was no way he could have heard my voice coming from the third floor. He knew he should come and see if I was all right. Miles got up and got dressed, then came up to my door and knocked. It seemed to me that his knock came just after I had answered "*Yes*" to Yehovah. I quickly got up, wondering who could possibly be knocking at my door so early. It was Miles!

"***I heard you calling my name***," he said to me while standing in the hallway.

I tried to make sense of what he was saying, while aware that our conversation might wake up others in neighboring rooms.

"No. That's ridiculous!

But even if I was… how could you hear me?" I loudly whispered. ***"I am on the third floor, and you are on the first!"***

"I did!" declared Miles.

"***You'd better come in!***" I said.
It was all so strange, and before I knew it, I found myself saying to Miles:
"I have just told Yehovah that I would marry you!"

UNEXPECTED

Miles had been shocked but very, very happy when I told him of my agreement with Yehovah to marry him. He had often thought that if I was ever going to marry him, it would take divine intervention, and that is exactly what happened!

Of course, no one expected to have a wedding take place at Mount Sinai, least of all us! When Miles broke the news at the breakfast table that morning, everyone was delighted! I think I was in a daze that day as I do not remember much of it.

We had one evening and one day to prepare. We met that evening with a small group - Pastor Art, who would officiate at the wedding, Janice and David, Jenny, Roland and Lilian, and Patrick. Miles and I shared the supernatural events of the night hours.

We remembered the Ketubah ceremony Yehovah ordained at Mount Sinai (Exodus 19) was a wedding covenant. In fact, the Jewish wedding ceremony is based on those events that took place at Mount Sinai around 3500 years ago. It included a chuppah (covering) to represent the cloud covering and presence of the God of Abraham, Isaac and Jacob, and a Ketubah - the written agreement setting out the terms of the covenant. Janice suggested that this occasion would be the perfect time for the team to stand together before Yehovah and make our own oath of obedience to Him. Our gathered friends asked if Miles and I would be willing to share our Ketubah ceremony with the whole team, representing all those who would be the bride of the Messiah. Without hesitation and in unison Miles and I said, ***"Yes!"***

And so, the wedding planning began, starting with Jenny, Janice and I earnestly praying that Yehovah would provide a cloud as a chuppah (cover) – just as He had so many centuries before for the children of Israel in the wilderness, when He spoke to Israel from the mountain. [The Saudi Arabian government severely frowns on bringing anything Jewish / Hebraic into the country or to the mountain, so no one had brought with them a prayer shawl, that could otherwise have been a bridal cover for me.]

"Torah is often referred to as a marriage agreement,
and with their acceptance of the
commandments they became the 'bride.'
This sets in motion the rest of the biblical narrative
of how a loving God seeks to restore His wandering bride.
And it is through the renewing of this covenant
in the death, burial, and resurrection of Yeshua
that we have finally found peace and restoration with Yehovah.
And I thank Yah that this covenant is no longer
written on tables of stone, but now it is written on our hearts."
Author unknown

The day before the wedding would be the team's second day at Mount Sinai. With this being the one and only day to prepare for all matters of marriage, I decided not to go, but stay at the hotel. This was the decision of Pastor Art, Janice and Jenny too. So while the other members of the expedition were climbing rocks, finding inscriptions, taking photos and filming, Janice and Jenny busied themselves writing out individual copies of the Ketubah – a written agreement - for each one of us in our team. It was a tremendous labor of love and commitment, as each handwritten copy took a good length of time! In the Ketubah, they carefully outlined the information found in Exodus and Deuteronomy about the covenant and Yehovah's promises to those who obeyed from the heart.

Pastor Art and I met for some pre-wedding counsel, then while he prepared his thoughts and notes for the ceremony, I was faced with the big question every girl has for her wedding day… What was I going to wear? My options were limited. In fact, did I even have any options other than my climbing clothes? Ah… no. Yet even if I had, it would not have been permitted to wear any bridal attire at Mount Sinai in Saudi Arabia.

For the remainder of my day, I prayed and tried to rest. The antidote to the nervousness I felt, was to revise my conversation with Yehovah - ***"Will you trust Me?"*** and my response, ***"Yes."***

The evening meal for our team was at the best local restaurant in town, where we had eaten a number of meals together. Our last meal here was the evening after climbing the mountain. Our conversations that night were energized and animated as we shared our varying and incredible experiences of that day. And now tonight, at our pre-wedding evening meal, we were once again in high spirits as we anticipated tomorrow's ceremony on Mount Sinai - the Mountain of God. All would attend. Tomorrow, I would become Mrs. Cate Jones!

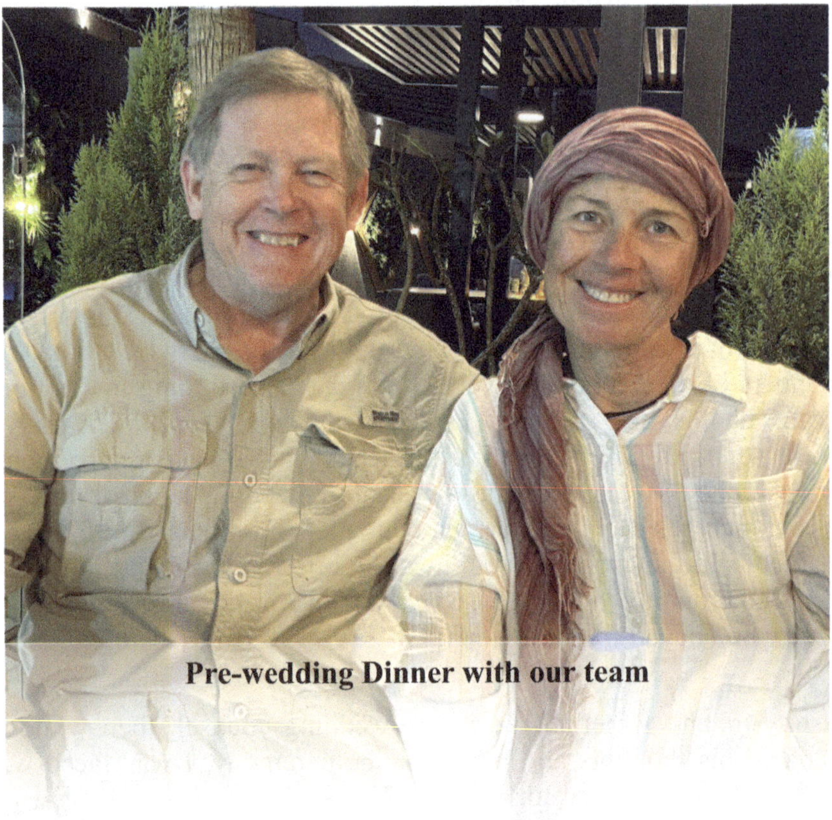

Pre-wedding Dinner with our team

It so happened, that in the same restaurant that evening was Pastor Steve Cioccolanti from Australia (now USA). He and his wife had just arrived to visit Mount Sinai. Having heard that Dr. Jones and the team were in the restaurant, Pastor Steve came to our table during dinner to chat and exchange contact details. Tomorrow, he would be on the other side of the mountain at the Split Rock while we would be at Moses' Altar.

THE WEDDING

"…be ready on the third day"
Exodus 19:11

On March 14th 2023, I woke in my Haql hotel room realizing the magnitude of the day that was before me. I was getting married, when just two days prior it wasn't even a thought in my mind. And we were about to be married on Mount Sinai at Moses' Altar, beneath the cleft in the rock and Elijah's Cave. How does one process that?

With a badly sprained wrist, I showered and washed my hair as best as I could. This was not easy, or fast! In hindsight, I should have asked one of my sisters to at least help me get my clothes on, dry my hair, and assist me with packing. We would make our final departure from the hotel after breakfast.

I dressed in my climbing khaki pants, white linen shirt and climbing boots. On my head I would wear a wine colored scarf that Lilian would help me with before we got to Moses' Altar. I would also wear the Esther belt. It had dawned on me yesterday why Renae had been led by the Holy Spirit to have me bring this Esther belt to Saudi Arabia. What had she said to me?

"There is a special purpose for you with this.
I don't know what it is, but you will find out."

Surely, it was *for such a time as this, I thought!* I was getting married to Miles and we were all going to renew our covenant vows of marriage to Yehovah, The King, at His Holy Mountain! My heart was filling with quiet wonder at what was about to take place.

Breakfast was once again served to the team in the lobby of hotel. I had no appetite but I forced myself to eat something small. As we left in our convoy of Land Cruisers, the sun shone bright in a clear blue sky, and just like every other day, it was hot and dry. Once more, we were making the three-and-a-half-hour journey to the mountain. This time, I traveled separately from Miles. I was in a Land Cruiser with

Janice, who would be my matron of honor, and Lilian, who would help with my headscarf. Miles traveled with Roland, who would be his best man, and Patrick his cameraman. This was the last day for us to be at Mount Sinai. It was Tuesday.

Miles was also wearing his pants, shirt and boots which were his daily expedition wear throughout our days in Saudi Arabia. Today though, for the wedding, he had decided not to wear his Indiana Jones hat. Later he regretted this as his face was badly sunburned.

Our convoy of Land Cruisers arrived at the mountain. Since this was the last day we would be on this research trip, we had asked if our Saudi drivers would give us privacy for our final gathering together at the Mountain. We had all been careful to not inform them that we were performing a wedding ceremony, as we did not want to have this stopped or interrupted. Our drivers therefore stayed with the Land Cruisers.

Lilian helped me to fix my head scarf and place the Esther belt on me. The sash's soft wine color matched my headscarf. Lilian had wrapped the fabric twice around my waist, and the bell ends hung low on the side of my body. The delicate sound of the small gold bells made me feel feminine and beautiful for my wedding day! Could there be any better reason for wearing the Esther belt than this day, I wondered. But of course. This is what it was for - a wedding at Sinai!

Our expedition team made our way to Moses' Altar. As we did, some of the team foraged for wild grasses that would be my wedding bouquet. It was to be a perfect wedding bouquet!

At Moses' Altar with the twelve pillars that had represented the twelve tribes of Israel, we set up cameras and phones and found the best places to stand and film. For me, and I'm sure for others too, I felt a holy reverence and awe in my heart for what we were about to be a part of. It was a quiet expectation. We had even decided beforehand; it was only right that we would stand before Yehovah at His Holy Mountain with our shoes off. Without a doubt, we were on holy ground! There was great joy in our hearts and on our faces.

For some reason, not all of our team had made it to where we were at Moses' Altar. What had happened to them, we wondered. Instead of our full head count, there was only Miles and I, Pastor Art, and 12 others. Really? We had exactly 12 witnesses, correlating to the remnants of the twelve pillars of the twelve tribes of Israel where we now stood. This of course had not been planned. We were to later reflect that it is no light thing to serve the Creator of the Universe, who is the God of Abraham, Isaac, Jacob, Moses and Yeshua. Of the thirty-plus original tour members only fifteen took part in our ceremony. Half went home a week earlier, and others missed this wedding ceremony for mysterious or even inexplicable reasons.

Wide-eyed at the thought of 12 witnesses, someone then noticed a cloud hovering near the top of Mount Sinai. We were even more excited! Yehovah had heard our request for a chuppah, a bridal cover.

Miles and I, along with Janice and Roland either side of us, positioned ourselves. Pastor Art began the wedding ceremony. I was somewhat nervous, but the more overwhelming emotion was definitely wonder and awe. Was this really happening? I was just a woman from New Zealand, who just happened to flee domestic violence and find a safe house in Kerrville, Texas, who just happened to meet Dr. Miles Jones at a restaurant one night, who just happened to be a biblical archeologist and researcher, who just happened to be leading an expedition to Mount Sinai, who just happened to be standing before me now on Mount Sinai before twelve witnesses, who just happened to be speaking his wedding covenant vows to me, while there just happened to be one solitary cloud over our heads!

I remembered my dream two months prior where Yehovah spoke to my heart saying, "***There is more ahead of you than time would suggest Fiona.***" Wasn't that the truth! Since that time, I had been saying, "*Hineini. Here I am. I am ready Yehovah.*" And now, *here I was*, before The King! There was no 'pause' button I could press to let this all sink in.

We had prepared our hearts and our minds to receive what Yehovah had in store for us. Though none of us had anticipated a wedding and a covenant ceremony with Yehovah, we had begun our preparations long before we arrived, in fasting, and prayer and diligently seeking to better know Yehovah and Yeshua in His Word and through prayer. Some of us had fasted and prayed for three days in preparation, as Esther did before appearing before the King. After all, our first visit to Yehovah's Holy Mountain had coincided with Purim!

And now, as Miles lovingly nudged me, I once again heard the delicate sound of the bells on the Esther belt. What was it Renae had said about the belt?

"It's worn to bring the essence of Yah's presence
where He desires dominion.
It's a tangible visual, that changes the atmosphere
through His Presence and His Directives.
It is only to be worn when He directs, and for His purposes."

I believe the Spirit of Esther ***- to rise up and do what you are made to do in the name of Yehovah -*** was with me there at Mount Sinai. Yehovah had given me a new repaired heart - a heart of full capacity to live out His purposes. Yehovah had certainly given Esther such a heart, to rise up and do what He made her to do in His name! Now, the Spirit of Yehovah was rising up within me to accomplish and fulfill His plan and purpose. I too was born for such a time as this.

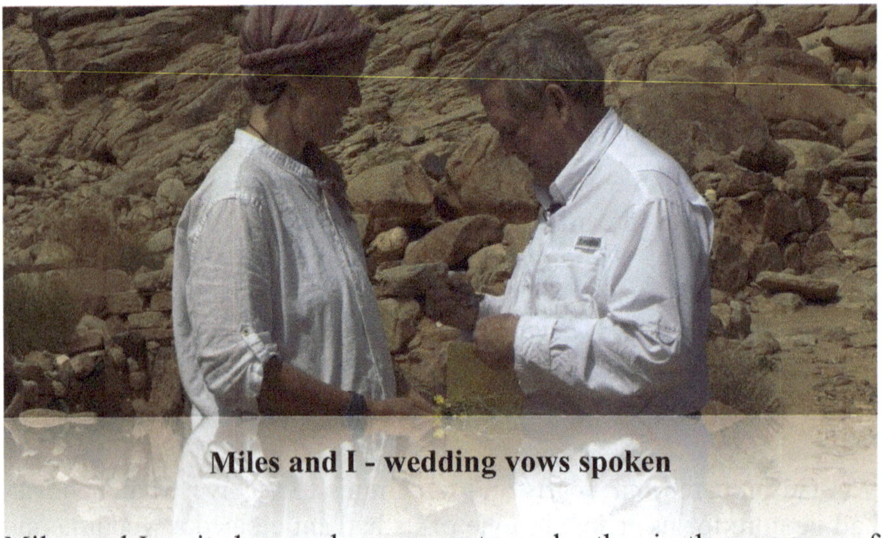

Miles and I - wedding vows spoken

Miles and I recited our solemn vows to each other in the presence of Yehovah, Yeshua and Israel i.e. our brothers and sisters present, who like us were grateful ingrafts to Yehovah's covenant people through faith in Yeshua. We too, are now called the children of Israel. And so we were pronounced husband and wife.

Pronounced husband and wife before Yehovah

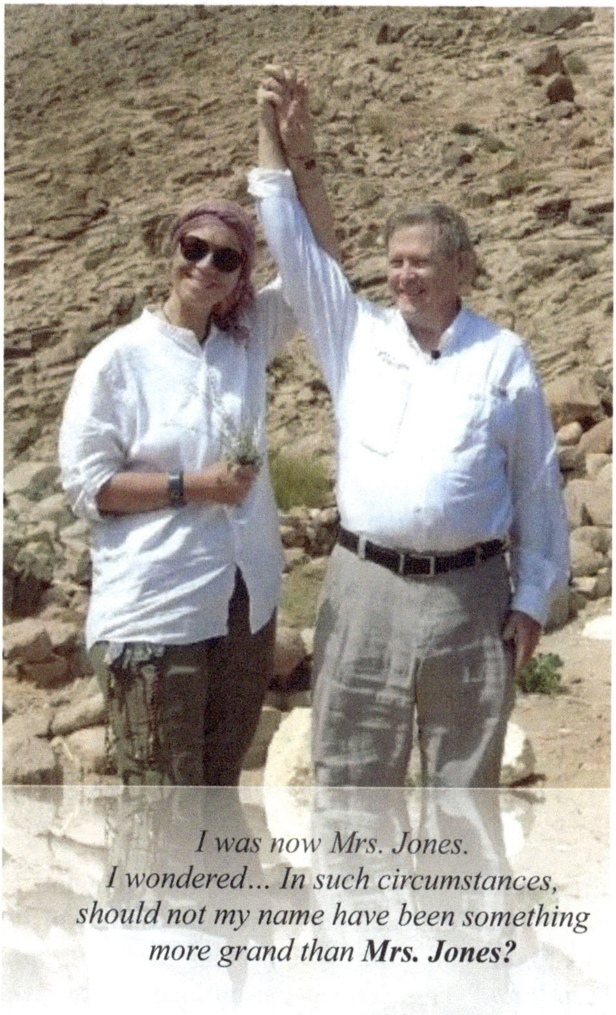

I was now Mrs. Jones.
I wondered... In such circumstances, should not my name have been something more grand than ***Mrs. Jones?***

Pastor Art turned to address all of us who were humbly gathered, to begin the second part of the covenant ceremony. He led us all in confession of our sins, repentance, and our asking Yehovah's forgiveness, prior to partaking of the communion of crackers and juice. This we did in remembrance of Yeshua giving His life on our behalf, redeeming us by His own blood (Luke 22:19-20).

[We were later to wonder if this covenant meal, in remembrance of Yeshua, broke the curse of the golden calf worship - Exodus 32!]

"See, the days are coming," declares Yehovah,
"when I shall make a renewed covenant with the house of Israel
and with the house of Judah, *not like the covenant I made*
with their fathers in the day when I strengthened their hand
to bring them out of the land of Mitsrayim,
My covenant which they broke, though
I was a husband to them," declares Yehovah.
"For this is the covenant I shall make
with the house of Israel after those days, declares Yehovah:
I shall put My Torah in their inward parts,
and write it on their hearts.
And I shall be their God, and they shall be My people."
Jeremiah 31:31-33

For many centuries, Jewish weddings took place on the third day of the week, to remember that they prepared for three days to meet Yehovah at the Mountain. They marry beneath a canopy – called a chuppah – in remembrance of the covering of clouds at Mount Sinai. On the third day, as part of the covenant ceremony, Yehovah spoke to the people from the mountain, beginning with the ten commandments (see Exodus 20:1-17).

THE WRITTEN KETUBAH

Pastor Art turned to the people gathered at the altar and read from Exodus, and as part of that ceremony, we committed to do all that Yehovah told us to do. Three times we proclaimed, "***All that Yehovah has said, we shall do***." This echoed the momentous occasion of the covenant first presented over 3500 years ago to the children of Israel in Exodus 19:5-6.

So Moses came and called for the elders of the people,
and laid before them all these words which Yehovah commanded him.

Then all the people gathered that day answered and said,
"All that Yehovah has spoken we will do."
Exodus 19:7-8

So Moses came and told the people
all the words of Yehovah and all the judgments.

Once more, those who gathered there said with one voice,
"All the words which Yehovah has said we will do."

Then he (Moses) took the Book of the Covenant
and read in the hearing of the people.

A third time they said, ***"All that Yehovah has said we will do,***
and be obedient."
Exodus 24:3-7

This was the first covenant to be made at The Mountain of God since the time Moses and the children of Israel came together. We, now also children of Israel, once again said ***three "I do's,"*** and so renewing our wedding vows with Yehovah. Even more significant, was that we were the first New Covenant believers who had made a Ketubah with Yehovah at Mt. Sinai!

At the conclusion of the ceremony, we signed our Ketubahs. Each person requested signatures from the others. It was wonderful to see the zeal to complete the Ketubah witness! As we were all about to leave this incredible place and experience, I asked if I could speak the Aaronic Blessing over everyone present - and in Hebrew too, of course. As I did, I spoke with a boldness I had not possessed before.

With our hearts full to overflowing with praise and thanksgiving, we gathered up everything, and now for the last time we made our way back to our Land Cruisers where our Saudi drivers were taking a siesta. We had no idea that we were about to literally see how Yehovah *changes the atmosphere through His Presence and His Directives*!

In the third month after the children of Israel
had gone out of the land of Egypt,
on the same day, they came ... and camped there before the mountain.
And Moses went up to God, and Yehovah called to him from the
mountain, saying, "Thus you shall say to the house of Jacob,
and tell the children of Israel:
'You have seen what I did to the Egyptians,
and how I bore you on eagles' wings and brought you to Myself.

'Now therefore, if you will indeed obey My voice and keep My
covenant, then you shall be a special treasure to Me above all people;
for all the Earth is Mine.
And you shall be to Me a kingdom of priests and a holy nation...
And Yehovah said to Moses, "Behold, I come to you in the
thick cloud, that the people may hear when I speak with you,
and believe you forever."
Then it came to pass on the third day, in the morning,
that there were ***thunderings and lightnings,***
and a thick cloud on the mountain*;... Now Mount Sinai was*
completely in smoke, because Yehovah descended upon it in fire.
Its smoke ascended like the smoke of a furnace...
Exodus 19:1-9,16,18

Once we were all back to the Land Cruisers, our Saudi guides brought out food. We sat on the surrounding scattered rocks to eat. For Miles and I we were eating our first meal together as husband and wife. Even this was to prove memorable beyond belief.

Heavy thunderclouds were starting to replace the small puffy white cloud, as we walked back from Moses' Altar. But then we had barely been able to finish eating our meal when it began to sprinkle and a powerful wind arose, blowing dark clouds into the area. We felt a sprinkle of rain, as we began to see ever darkening thunder clouds moving in toward the blackened peak of Mount Sinai. The wind took Miles' hat off and threatened to do the same with my plate, but I clutched it tighter in my hands trying to eat what I could of my meal. But that was not to happen either - the great wind blew ever harder!

I was so enthralled with what I was seeing, hearing and feeling, that I ran to Janice and began to sing, "*How great is Yehovah (our God), sing with me how great is Yehovah (our God), and all will see how great, how great is Yehovah (our God).*" Janice was quick to join me in praise. We were truly amazed, and as we sang our hearts out together to Yehovah, while at the same time we each were videoing all that was before us.

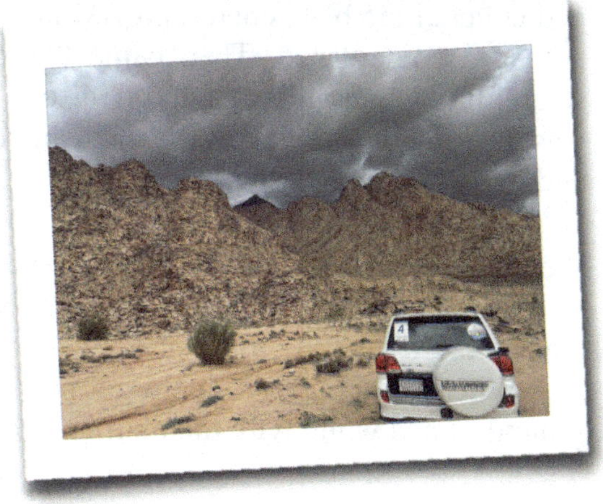

The dark thunder clouds were now completely covering the top of Mount Sinai – just as the clouds had covered it when Yehovah spoke from the cloud to the people below, proclaiming the covenant to them. Yehovah was giving a clear sign that He heard our voices! But He wanted to make sure there was no doubt. His celestial miracles were only beginning.

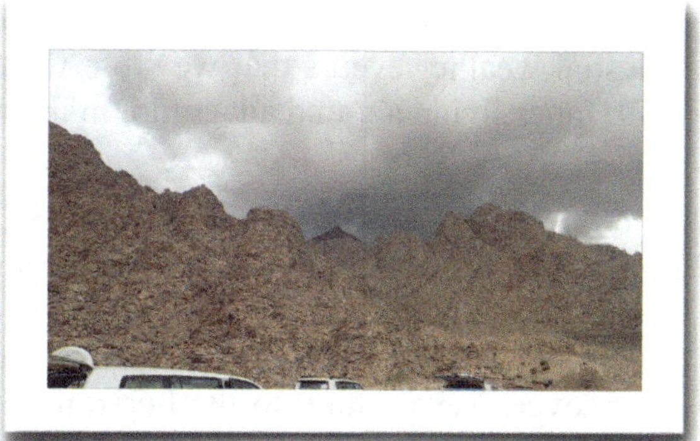

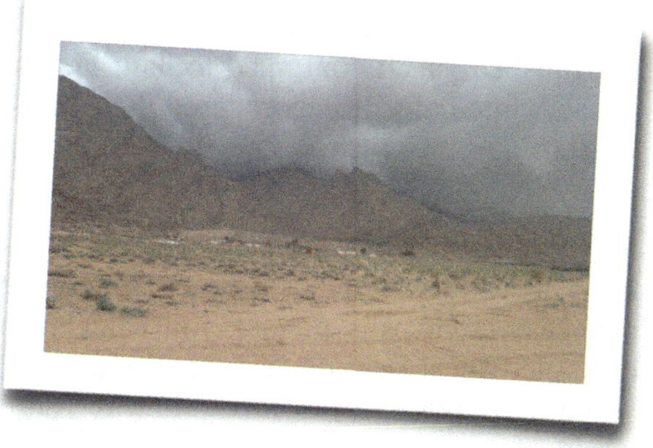

Lightning and thunder came closer and closer. The clouds grew darker

"Thunderings and lightnings, and a thick cloud on the mountain"

and covered the blackened top of Mount Sinai! We KNEW this could not be a coincidence. Then came the rain! It was then we started scrambling to get into the Land Cruisers. The rain became a deluge! It was the kind of torrent that the windshield wipers cannot keep up with and it did not relent.

We were rejoicing at this miracle! We were in a desert that receives less than an inch of rain each year. The water fell so hard and so fast that even after getting into our Land Cruisers, the drivers could barely see! When we thought it could get no worse, it began to hail and the ground turned white with the marble-sized hail!

Miles and I were in our own Land Cruiser with a driver. We were, after all, the newlyweds! I was overwhelmed not only by these celestial weather events that we were witnessing, but that I was now Mrs. Jones living a grand adventure in the wilderness of Sinai!

Our drivers had difficulty dealing with the conditions. They desperately wanted to get out of there before getting hopelessly mired in the flooded roadway which had been graded but not yet paved at this stage. The day had blackened like nightfall as the storm clouds now covered everything to the horizon. This weather was something extreme and unexpected for them to be dealing with.

We were all exuberant as we drove to the camp. Still, Yehovah was not finished yet. It continued to hail. For as far as the eye could see, small, white balls of hail covered the earth – looking as if the ground was covered in manna!

Yehovah had already prepared the footsteps of each of our lives to bring us to this moment in time. He knew every single one of them and His timing was precise and calculated. There was yet another example of just how precise His timing was. Janice's husband David asked her, "*What day is this?*" It was Tuesday. The third day of the week. Then he asked, "*How many times have we been here?*" Janice said, "*This is the third day!*"

We came to realize another wonder-filled thing, that not only was it the third occasion our team had been at Mount Sinai, but we were at

Mount Sinai renewing our vows on the **<u>third day</u>** of the week - as per Exodus 19:11! As a matter of fact, we were in the camp of the children of Israel! The only thing that would have made this event more powerful was to hear the voice of Yehovah! But the ever louder booming of thunder and the bright crackling of lightning all around us, was this not the voice of Yehovah? Had we not heard the voice of the shofar on the mountain as well?

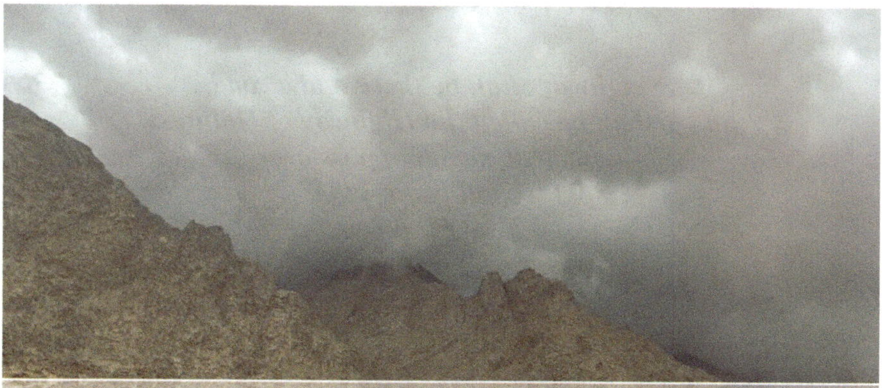

Then it came to pass on the third day, in the morning,
that there were thunderings and lightnings,
and a thick cloud on the mountain;
and the sound of the trumpet was very loud,
so that all the people who were in the camp trembled.
Exodus 19:16

At this point, Janice and I were frantically trying to call each other from our respective cars as we knew that Yehovah was performing a MASSIVE MIRACLE for us. But our cell phone service had failed! So, when our cars aligned, we put our windows down and shouted to each other above the noise of the hail, "***HE heard us! HE heard us!***"

We were all laughing and marveling at what we were experiencing and seeing. A great testimony of Yehovah moving in his people. Was it possible that ancient portal of Psalm 24 could manifest in modern times? Psalm 24 did call it an *eternal portal* opened upon Har Yehovah through which the Almighty does come through as He chooses. As if our minds weren't blown enough! We came down from The Mountain and danced with the Arabs in the rest area beside the road. Everyone was astounded. It almost never rains like this in Arabia.

Later I was to reflect on the dream I had on February 14, 2023, where a selection of different shades of blue linens were put before me and I was to choose one, and then seeing the word ISAIAH. I wondered if the deluge of rain was to be symbolic of a Mikva, or baptism - that we, His bride, were being purified?

A highway shall be there and a road,
and it shall be called the Highway of Holiness.
The unclean shall not pass over it,
but it shall be for others.
Isaiah 35:8

To go home and tell the story of what happened that day may not be believed, except that we had filmed and photographed everything of the ceremony and of these extreme celestial weather events. And now, as our time in Saudi Arabia and at Har Yehovah was drawing to a close, we headed back to Tabuk for our final night, and this brought about a change in plan.

The Millennium Hotel, the hotel we had stayed in on our arrival to Saudi Arabia and were to return to now for our final night, was no longer available to us due to the weather events. This was because the government's thousands of NEOM workers had to abandon their work and seek shelter. All of the shifts of workers required housing till there could be a return to work. The government seconded the Millennium Hotel, which meant we had to find an alternative hotel. This was to be a blessing in disguise too, as another hotel was found that was even nicer. Well at least for Miles and I it was, as we were given the honeymoon suite, complete with a Jacuzzi! Had someone other than Yehovah organized this for us? It didn't appear so. No one seemed to have any idea how it happened! At least no one confessed.

The great storm from Mount Sinai followed us to Tabuk, where we drove through flooded streets. Yet as the storm raged outside our hotel, Miles and I were unaware. I am thinking we were excused for having other things on our mind. And it had been a momentous day!

At 3:00 am the next morning we were loading our luggage into the Land Cruisers for the final time. From Tabuk we made the hour and a half flight to the airport in Jeddah, from where we caught another back to the States. Having boarded the plane in Tabuk to fly to Jeddah, a Saudi Arabian man shared photos and video of the snow that had fallen at Mount Sinai, Jabal al-Lawz only hours before, and which had begun to fall soon after we had left. Yehovah continued with great wonders! A deluge of rain, hail and now snow! Yehovah continued to proclaim through the storm that he heard his children's vows.

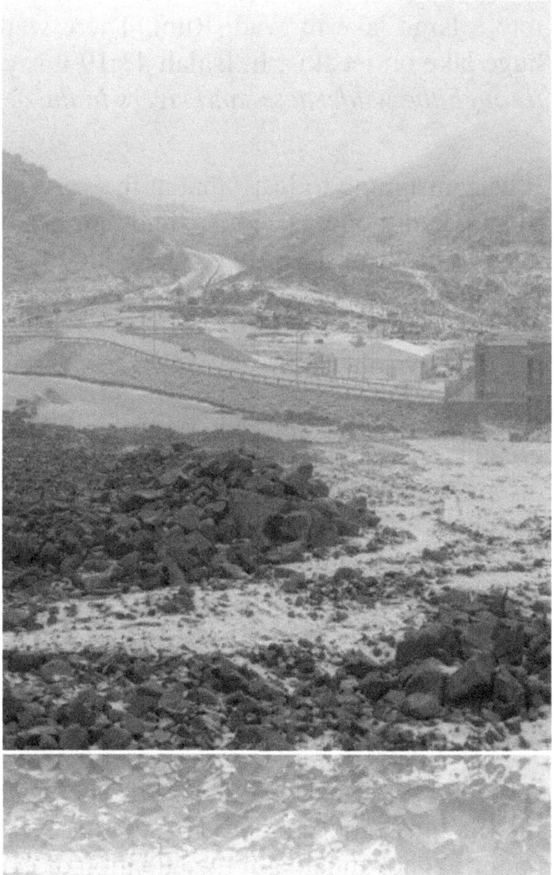

The snow that fell on Mount Sinai, Jabal al-Lawz 14th March 2023

We were soon to discover other things once back home.

On the day of our marriage at Sinai, March 14, 2023, in the south of Arabia, there was a monumental flood. That weather started in the north of Arabia with the Ketubah ceremony at Sinai. Remember that Saudi Arabia was entering into summer at that time, temperatures above 100 degrees Fahrenheit. That year, during the first weeks of the summer season there was flooding, hail and heavy snow across the region. In Tabuk, Riyadh and Jeddah they were digging out of the snow. There was incredible flooding over much, if not most, of Arabia and Israel. There was flooding in Oman. There was flooding in Yemen. There was flooding in the Negev Desert of Israel. Rivers of snow and ice water began flooding through the cities of Arabia!

Three weeks before our arrival, a geyser had erupted in the Rub' al Khali in the south. It created an incredible flowing river that gathered into a large lake in Wadi Rum. There were people riding across this huge lake on jet skis. In Isaiah 43:19 it says, "*I will even build a road through the wilderness, and rivers in the desert.*"

It was intriguing to learn that at the very same time we were at Mount Sinai when the rains, floods, and hail began, Pastor Steve Cioccolanti and his group were on the other side of the mountain, at Split Rock! He recorded video of what they saw and experienced of the extreme weather events.

And as you can imagine, these extreme weather events captured a great deal of attention around the world. In fact, members of our team discovered that the typical rainfall in the Tabuk Region of Saudi Arabia is approximately 33.5mm (1.32″) each year. It appears the average yearly number was exceeded in only a few minutes on March 14, 2023, the day of our covenant ceremony! In the south of Arabia, massive amounts of rain fell within a few hours. Roads and bridges were washed away. The streets became rivers and washed away even the large trucks that tried to cross them.

Little did we know that these extreme weather events would continue for months and spread to all parts of Arabia and the entire region. Yehovah had got the attention of every man, woman, and child in Saudi Arabia. We started to wonder if the storm could be symbolic of Yehovah cleansing us? Would it be a biblical symbol of the outpouring of the Holy Spirit as described in the book of Joel? The outpouring of rain as given in Scripture is given as a symbol of the outpouring of Yehovah's Spirit. Even as I write this a year later (2024) it is reported that the sands of Arabia where we had been, are covered with green grass.

Isaiah 35:7,8 and Isaiah 41:18,20 are fulfilled. Isaiah 43:19-21 and 44:1-4 are both in the midst of happening. In the past months fountains are springing forth in the Desert of Saudi Arabia. Water flows once more at Mount Sinai. The almond trees on Mount Sinai have blossomed. The Euphrates is nearly dry. These are incredible and awe-inspiring times we are living in! The call is to repent and return. To Teshuvah. As Yehovah called Israel to return in its last days before judgement, He is now calling all people. All nations.

Finally...

"It is hard for our modern minds to comprehend
the possibility that behind remarkable events in the world,
could lie a deeper story, of an unseen Hand.
Remove any of the events leading up to them,
the twists and the quirks, or move any of them out of place,
and none of it would have come out exactly as it did.
Had we not... had I not... had they not... had this not...
And yet it is not so much that the mystery works inside
the parameters of human history: it is that human history
works inside the parameters of the mystery."

Jonathan Cahn - *Josiah Manifesto*

What happened for me at Mount Sinai has been an incredible part of my story to write. A mystery to unveil. A putting together of the pieces. It could be considered by some to just be a random lot of events and happenings that all strangely lined up. However, I believe nothing was of happenstance or accidental, and that Yehovah's plans and purposes were brought together in a spectacular way. He lined all things up and provided numerous 'signature cards'. What Yehovah did at Mount Sinai was with phenomenal prowess!

Chief Editor's comment: *This has reminded me of your smashed up 1000-piece jigsaw puzzle, and gave me an image of all these events being pieces in the grand puzzle of your life, and in a way that only Yehovah can do, He is rightly piecing it all back together for you.*

And this a picture of all our lives really - the myriad of ways Yehovah's hand is orchestrating all things to be fitted together in His perfect plan and timing, even the bringing together of all the people involved in this mountain, whether they have been physically there, or helped in some way to make ***this place*** *and* ***His name upon it*** *known (like editors, even).*

A man's heart plans his way, but Yehovah directs his steps.
Proverbs 16:9

Of all the people in the world Yehovah could have chosen to be married at His mountain, He chose Miles and me. Why? We know that Yehovah spoke to ancient Israel through prophetic acts. Not all the prophetic acts were understood at the time. Perhaps all that happened to us was, or is, to happen without any knowledge of the prophetic significance on our part. It is simply enough that it was Yehovah's purpose.

Yet I am wondering if the experience I had at Har Yehovah might be to unravel a mystery that would bring not only understanding and healing to my own heart but understanding and healing to the hearts of many.

On the morning of February 29, 2024, Renae called me with great excitement in her voice. A revelation had risen up in her that morning as she had come out of her prayer closet and was walking across her kitchen floor. The revelation was this, that in all the world, Yehovah chose me, He ordained me to be there at His Holy Mountain. That He wanted to marry me there. Yes, I had married Miles, and yes those of our group also pledged and signed the Ketubah, but He had chosen me to be the bride.

And Moses said to the people, ***[Earnestly] remember this day in which you came out from Egypt, out of the house of bondage and bondmen, for by strength of hand Yehovah brought you out from this place.***
Exodus 13:3 AMPC

After all the devastation in my life, Yehovah showed me that my life counts. And that just as Moses instructed the Israelites to *"earnestly remember...",* I too was to *earnestly remember* that Yehovah had brought me out of bondage, and that by His strength of hand, He brought me out from there. It was as if Yehovah said to me, "*I'll tell you who you are — I'll put you on My holy mountain as a bride! - no longer wounded, abandoned, rejected. I am your husband!*" Mount Sinai was to heal my heart. It was to tell me - **let go of the old me. Do not be bound by your past. Let it go. Will you be Mine? Free of everything that has gone before.**

This is the biblical mystery of the bride and groom! In the beginning was God, and God is love. And so before there was anything else, there was love. We were *made* for love! The events that played out were a love story between Yehovah and *me*. A phenomenal love story! What a romance this was, on March the 14th, 2023 for the Kingdom of God. I should never doubt it. I am of the bridegroom's house, and I am in covenant! He is my story from beginning to end. He is the author of my faith and the finisher of my story. All my life experiences are in Yehovah's hands. As Renae said to me, "*this is the time for you to get on the horse and ride with Him!*"

Our Ketubah ceremony at Mount Sinai was the first, since Moses. Perhaps the last! The Saudis will now zealously guard the groups at the mountain to make sure such religious ceremonies do not happen. Our Sovereign God brought us to His Mountain as the last expedition to cross the desert in our Land Cruisers. In the 10 days we were there, they were building the nearby city of NEOM so fast that we had gone to The Mountain across the desert and were leaving The Mountain that day on paved roads. Everything from that point forward would be tightly regulated, even though many more people would be allowed to visit The Mountain.

It turned out that our agenda for the trip was one thing. Yehovah's purpose was another. *We were in the right place at the right time, doing what He had called us to do...* ***"for such a time as this"*** (Esther 4:14). We were on Yehovah's program. Truly amazing. Such a coup was Yehovah's planning. All that had happened on our journey to Mount Sinai was above and beyond all I could have imagined and hoped for.

2024 Looking Back:
Like the Israelites in bondage while in Egypt, Yehovah *did* hear me groaning in anorexia, depression and suicidality. Yehovah *did* bring me out from under the oppression of Jack and the Cruel Master and freed me. Yehovah *did* rescue me from marital and psychiatric abuse, with His powerful arm. I *did* know that it was Yehovah my God, who took me to my Red Sea Road, and brought me through a wilderness experience. And I *do* know that it was Yehovah who eventually brought me to the land He solemnly swore to give to Abraham, Isaac, and Jacob, and that He *has* given to me the Promised Land as my own possession. (Exodus 6:5-8)

I have other thoughts and wonderings about this Mount Sinai experience, and I expect even more will come, but I conclude with this:

Just as Moses was born for such a time… to deliver the Israelites from bondage, and just as Esther was born for such a time… to save her people from annihilation… *you and I were born with a God-ordained destiny* for our lives.

While Satan will try everything under the sun to keep you and I from our destiny, ***the Word of Yehovah*** and ***His divine Presence*** are the ***roadmap*** to that destiny.

Let us all rise to that for which Yehovah placed us in our mother's womb***… for such a time as this!***

*****

Epilogue: Song of the Sea

The Song of Moses and Israel

Then Moses and the children of Israel
sang this song to Yehovah, singing,

"I will sing to the Lord, for He has triumphed gloriously;
The horse and its rider He has thrown into the sea."
Exodus 15:1 (CJB)

When I left New Zealand on my *Red Sea Road*, I had no answers and I could not see the way, but Yehovah *parted the waves* for me, just as He did for the Israelites… He saved me from destruction!

And just as Moses and the Israelites sang a song to Yehovah in celebration of their freedom from Egyptian slavery and the destruction of the Egyptian army (see *Song of the Sea*, or, *Song of Moses* in Exodus 15:1b-18), the writing of this book is my personal '***Song of the Sea***', written to express *my* gratitude and praise for Yehovah's deliverance and victory over my enemies - over Satan - and to acknowledge Yehovah's providential lovingkindness to me.

*****

It has now been 15 years since 2010 - when my heart was ripped out. The abuse and trauma of over two decades might have, and nearly did, finish me. *How could I go on?*

As it was for the Israelites, there were extremely difficult days ahead for me. **In the long initial time of shock and loss, I did not think I could live another *hour*, let alone another day, week, month or year! I could not make the pain go away, and it constantly threatened to overtake me.**

The grief was so overwhelming, and the losses so catastrophic and excruciatingly painful. I knew it was indeed possible to die of a broken heart! But for Yehovah…

Yehovah's promise was that He would not leave me - that I would never walk alone. In my soul's unrelenting anguish, Yeshua drew so close to my broken heart and showed me His love and compassion in a myriad of ways.

Over and over, He reminded my soul: *I AM with you, I AM faithful, I will go before you, I will be behind you. I will provide. I will defend you. I will heal you. I will restore! Trust Me to bring you through.* ***I AM*** *can make a way where there seems to be no way!*

As best as I could, I held onto hope rather than despair - believing that healing and restoration *was* ahead. All my eggs were in one basket - My Heavenly Father's basket! Who else did I have?

Now, all these years later, I get to declare, *"I'm still alive!" "I did stop crying!" "I didn't lose my sanity!"* and *"Here I am now living on the other side of the world in Texas, having remarried at Mt. Sinai—Yehovah's Holy Mountain!"* How on Earth did all this come about, except by Abba's grace and mercy?

It is a marvel! And I am thoroughly thankful.

Joseph's story (see Genesis chapters 37-50) continues to give me great hope and encouragement. Joseph was rejected and thrown into a pit by his brothers… sold into slavery… wrongly accused… imprisoned… and abandoned… Then, after many long years, was brought before a king. This ultimately led to Joseph fulfilling a very great purpose that those painful years had prepared him for. Years that would bring meaning to all the hardship and injustice he had experienced in his life.

In Genesis 50:20, Joseph's brothers came to him in Egypt for help. They did not know that this was their brother who they had treated so wrongfully. When they realized it was Joseph, they were - of course - afraid! Joseph's words to his brothers were profound. Though Joseph had the power to annihilate his brothers as payback for all the years of his affliction, instead he spoke these words to them:

But as for you, you meant evil against me;
but God meant it for good, *in order to bring it about*
as it is this day, to save many people alive.
Genesis **50:20**

I have tethered myself to this same ***50/20 vision*** that Joseph had, trusting that what Satan, and Jack, meant for evil and destruction in my life, *"God has meant it for good, in order to bring it about as it is this day,"* a testimony of deliverance, to help bring hope to those suffering mental and emotional anguish, and those who are trying to get through seriously difficult circumstances.

Throughout the Scriptures, it says, "Thus *says* Yehovah". In Hebrew the word *says* is ***Amar***. This word is a past tense, and it means that Yehovah has ***already said,*** and ***it is already done***. Therefore, we can put our complete trust and faith in the Word of God, because when Yehovah says something, it is as good as done - no if's or maybe's. So stand on the Word, hold to the Word, and be confident in it!

My hope and pray for this book - *Red Sea Road to Sinai* - and the book that will follow, gives you eyes to see that our loving Heavenly Father and Savior Yeshua, can make a way for you to hope and to carry on, even when your way ahead seems daunting or impossible. May He help you to believe, *He is faithful.* And when your heart is breaking, to still believe - *He is faithful. So faithful.* Abba-Yehovah is with you in the middle of your suffering and loss. He longs to redeem all of it for you, if you will allow Him.

Shalom and Shalom,

Cate Jones

P.S. Elle Holcomb has a great vocal album called ***Red Sea Road.***
I invite you to listen and allow the words of her songs to bless you!

Preview of Following Book

A Voice in the Wilderness

Cate's story continues where Chapter 11 ends, telling what happened in her ***11-wilderness-years*** before Mount Sinai.

'A Voice in the Wilderness' will reveal what led up to Cate fleeing New Zealand, and what it was like to leave everything and everyone familiar...to pick up the pieces of her life, find safety, and start over, while experiencing profound grief, loss, and trauma that comes with *extreme parental alienation.*

Questions like: *What made it possible for Cate to carry on living without her children? How did she find and experience healing for all her life's painful experiences? And what has since happened between her and her children, who are now adults*...will get answered.

Cate will also share what she has learned through her experience of extreme parental alienation and describe the real but irrational manifestations displayed by children with *Parental Alienation Syndrome (PAS)*. Most importantly, Cate will reveal the striking parallel between the rampant issue of parental alienation that exists in our societies today, and the rampant issue of spiritual alienation! *Yehovah is also an alienated Parent* whose heart grieves over His many alienated children.

Satan - the father of lies - has the sole goal of alienating us from others ***and*** alienating us all from our Creator - who is our loving, faithful and truthful Father. Cate will reveal how people today who are alienated from their Creator and Savior Yeshua, often manifest '*Spiritual Parental Alienation Syndrome'*.

Just as it will be Yehovah's grace that will lead Cate's three children home to her, their loving mother, it will be Yehovah's grace that will lead His alienated children home to Him.

Appendix 1: Kayla's Story

While I was at Ashburn Clinic, I came to know a young patient by the name of Kayla who suffered with an an eating disorder. She was seventeen years old. What follows is an online conversation that Kayla initiated on livejournal.com. Kayla shares her Ashburn Clinic experience. She was an Ashburn patient at the time. Validating responses then follow from others who had once been patients at Ashburn Clinic.

*****

https://nz-ed.livejournal.com6184.html

09 September 2008
Ashburn Clinic [comments by Kayla W]

Community meetings are held in the mornings, twice weekly… Many meetings involve verbal abuse of patients, beneath the euphemism of a 'challenge'. Needless to say, it was humiliating to be heavily criticized by the staff members for my binge/purging in front of that many people (as was done on the 6th March). I left the meeting feeling like a criminal and hating myself even more for my behavior.

…There is a complete lack of confidentiality, trust and safety within the [Ashburn] community. If staff members aren't outright sharing confidential details of patients illnesses with other members of the community, they are implying it in order to 'cover their tracks'. Things like the numerical details of other patients' weight, weight gain/loss, are openly discussed between staff and the community. I find this particularly unhelpful, so after xxx [my nurse] shared the details of another patient's BMI [body mass index], I politely asked him, one-on-one, if he would mind not discussing such things in front of me. I was told: *"I'm not going to wrap you in cotton wool"*, and that was that.

…The Ashburn Clinic violates a number of patient's rights under the Code of Health and Disability Services Consumer's Rights. Firstly, the right of respect. The following are quotes said either to me or to other patients there, during my stay:

"All anorexics are one-eyed and deaf-eared"
"Are you thick?"
"You can starve yourself to death for all I care!"
"You're a bully. No one wants you here."
"You're obviously trying to undermine the whole community."
"You're sick. You're really sick!" [said with disgust]
"You must have misheard." [On questioning about abusive comments]
"You are destructive to the other patients."
"I think we're trying to find a bad guy here". [When people start questioning the staff, this is generally the response]

These are very disrespectful, and in some cases downright abusive. As I have said, for the few people who do benefit, many more are damaged or hindered in their recovery.

Love, Kayla

*****

Below, are the responses to Kayla's Post:

Scarby on December 7th, 2009
Hi Kayla,
I agree with you in terms of the violation to privacy and the lack of respect... I was in for just one month and i was nearly destroyed by their approach.
Hope this finds you well.

Guineapig93 on December 25th, 2013
My opinion:
I certainly agree with what you've said, it can really mess people up and they come out a heck of a lot worse than when they went in.

Yep *"trying to find a bad guy"* is usually the response when the staff are questioned by the patient group. Private information relating to your treatment is yours alone but is often shared among the group which is very humiliating, and if you don't like it and disagree with it then you get told you have trust issues. The staff always back each other up and they have the power to make your life a misery. Also I found that some staff were very rude and seemed to enjoy placing restrictions on people for kicks. There was a lot of unprofessionalism amongst staff also, for example leaving medical records and private documents lying around, unsecured in open areas, and if you listened you could hear them talking about patients. They made errors in dispensing medication frequently, (it happened to me 3 times) and every 6 months they put out a report and one time it said that medication administration errors had increased by 200%! They definitely breach your rights. I laid 2 complaints with the HDC [Health and Disability Commission] in my time there. They think they're the best when they're not, and they think they're untouchable upon their thrones.

End of comments from Live Journal

*****

I, Cate, had known Kayla. We were patients together at Ashburn Clinic. Her polite, well-meaning and sincere words that she posted online, remind me of her intelligent mind, gentle soul, and quiet demeanor. Seventeen-year-old Kayla was a very beautiful girl who carried deep sadness.

Kayla had been legally committed to Ashburn. A family court judge was required to approve her release. Each month she would go to meet with the judge when he was at Ashburn - and time after time Kayla was told she would not be released. Finally, she found a way of escaping.

Kayla committed suicide on Saturday, November 15, 2008 - only two months after her post on Live Journal. I had left Ashburn Clinic only weeks before her death. It broke my heart to hear this tragic news of Kayla.

According to another patient's reporting on this, "*There was an escape and suicide attempt when I was there and when they brought her [Kayla] back, they put everyone in a circle in the room for them all to give her feedback. It was entirely negative, telling her she was selfish etc. I was shocked and the only one saying, 'I'm glad you're ok.' She went again and succeeded a couple of weeks later.*"

(https://www.reddit.com/r/dunedin/comments/15wvdmu/has_anyone_been_to_ashburn_clinic_dunedin/?rdt=35110)

*****

Appendix 2: Healing Prayer

This prayer came under the anointing of the Holy Spirit after I had finished reading **Chapter 11 'Red Sea Road'** *to Lisa Townley. I share it with the reader for your help and encouragement too, for whatever tests and trials you and your family are facing in your life.*

Lisa: Father, we humble ourselves before You Yehovah. We thank you for Your redemption given to Cate. Thank you that this book has a beautiful and powerful plan. That through it, lives will be transformed because You do not waste anything. You say **all** things are going to be for Your glory. It *will be* for Your glory. That for all the horrendous acts that Cate has gone through, You shall be glorified.

We ask You Holy Spirit to reveal everything that needs to be healed in her heart. Restore her soul. We release to You every toxic emotion. We receive that healing. We chose right now to receive the cleansing of our imagination screens with the blood of Yeshua so we can clearly see the truth. Holy Spirit we invite you to come to expose every part of her soul that needs healing, restoration and freedom. We turn to you Yeshua. Thank you that you are here.

Cate: I release to you the residual shame and embarrassment. Sadness of years, grief for toxicity placed on my children, and the confusion I had in those years. I repent for years where I refused to listen to Your Word that would have set me free. Listening to Satan's voice and not Yours. Thank you that when I did hear Romans 8:38-39, *it did* set me free, knowing that nothing could ever separate me from Your love. I remember hearing that verse again and how powerful it was! Thank you for taking these emotions, now. Wash me clean, restore my soul, and apply your love, forgiveness and truth over my life. Thank you that You would do this for me.

Lisa: Holy Spirit we now invite your love to come filling every recess of her soul, healing every wound from every violation. Every time that she was raped, manipulated, controlled, shamed and afraid. We receive Your love. I speak restoration and healing over her physical body, since every cell carries memory. And I reverse the violation that was done to this body in the name of Yeshua.

I cancel the assignment to destroy her. Every violation sexually, mentally, physically, even with her eating disorder that was because of the violations. So we reverse the curse and command LIFE over her physical body in every cell from the top of head to the soles of her feet. You Yehovah are the Giver of life. We speak healing and wholeness over her brain, mind, mouth, digestive system, sexual organs. We speak complete healing and wholeness in the name of Yeshua.

Yeshua, you went about doing good and healing everyone who was oppressed by the devil. And you sent out your disciples to heal the sick and raise the dead, cast out devils. So right now in the authority you give us, *Cate, do you receive healing in your body right now?* (Cate: *"yes"*). So we receive by faith that authority and we receive healing in her entire body right now. Every side effect that she has been experiencing because of the years of hell, we now command to cease and desist in the mighty name of Yeshua!

Every spirit of infirmity that has been sitting on her, influencing her, affecting her, in any way, we paralyze you and destroy your works and affects, and we command you to leave now in the name of Yeshua!

We cancel the assignment upon her children for any of the curses that were placed upon her. Any of the abuse that landed on her, that would continue to any of her generations. We say *"NO! It shall not continue!"* We lift off of all three of her children, grandchildren, siblings, nieces and nephews, cousins, family all around, her - the works of darkness, and we command every curse to be reversed. Every spell, hex, vex, to be destroyed in the name of Yeshua.

We receive the blessings of unity, of family, of healing, of wholeness, of life, in the name of Yeshua. Amen.

No weapon forged against Cate, or anyone in her family - any of her children, or grandchildren, or great grandchildren, or great-great-grandchildren, shall prosper. And every tongue that rises against her and her family, shall be put to shame, because Yehovah says, *"She is righteous. They are Mine. Yes, they are Mine."*

By the blood of Yeshua, we are made righteous. We receive the powerful blood of Yeshua and the promises that come with that. Abundant life. Yeshua, you say the enemy only comes to steal, kill and destroy, BUT… You get the last word! You have come to give life and that MORE abundantly. We receive that abundant life over Cate, and over ALL her family, in your name HalleluYAH! Amen

Cate: Yehovah, I thank you with absolutely certainty and conviction that while the enemy has come to steal, kill and destroy my life, that his work is completely trumped by what Yeshua has done in and over my life. Yeshua has come and given me LIFE in all its fullness. So, what the enemy meant for harm, You Yehovah are using it for good.

I praise You for Your rescue and remedy in my life and my family's life. I have and will continue to overcome. Blessed be the name of my Redeemer Yeshua. Amen

Come to Me, Yeshua, all you who labor and are heavy laden,
and I will give you rest. Take My yoke upon you and learn from Me,
for I am gentle and lowly in heart,
and you will find rest for your souls.
Matthew 11:28-29

For God, Yehovah, so loved the world that He gave His
only begotten Son, Yeshua, that whoever believes in Him
should not perish but have everlasting life.
John 3:16

So then ***faith comes by hearing, and hearing by the Word of God.***
Romans 10:17

Appendix 3: Dr. Miles Jones

Yehovah is doing a new thing, and miracles continue at Mount Sinai and in Saudi Arabia. I believe Yehovah is calling His people to Teshuvah - to repent and turn back to Him - and determine to do what He asks us to do, because of His very great love for us.

"Now it shall come to pass in the latter days
That Har Yehovah's (the mountain of the LORD's) house (of prayer)
Shall be established on the top of the mountains,
And shall be exalted above the hills;
And all nations shall flow to it.

Many people shall come and say,
"Come, and let us go up to Har Yehovah (the mountain of the LORD)
To the house (of prayer) of the God of Jacob;
He will teach us His ways,
And we shall walk in His paths."
For out of Zion shall go forth the Torah,
And the Word of Yehovah from Jerusalem.
Isaiah 2: 2-3

We are seeing prophecy being fulfilled! "*Behold! I will do a new thing. Now it shall spring forth. Shall you not know it? I will even make a road in the wilderness, and rivers in the desert!*" (Isaiah 43:19) We drove out of Mount Sinai on a newly paved road. We were perhaps the first to drive it except for the workers who made it. The river that erupted in the Rub'al-Khali is not the last. The massive flooding has turned dry wadis (stream beds) into rivers all over the Saudi Peninsula. "*Har Yehovah's house of prayer shall be established on the top of the mountains... and all nations shall flow to it!*" (Isaiah 2:2) The Mountain of God is a Temple, a house of prayer. It has been hidden for 3,500 years. Now it is open again.

We were not the only group on the mountain. People of all nations have already started to come. Soon there will be thousands of them coming in on tourist buses daily from the hotels built nearby on the main highway going to the new city of NEOM. Millions will come every year from all the nations of the world. Israelis have been to the mountain already. They will come from everywhere. Now that we know where the hidden mountain is located!

"*You are those who forsake Yehovah, who forget my holy mountain!*" (Isaiah 65:11) Those days are now over, the covenant on the mountain has been renewed, not only by our small group - but soon by millions of believers. The Mountain of Yehovah has even been hidden in Scripture. There are various names for the mountain; Har Horeb, Har Sinai, Har Elohim, BUT **Har Yehovah** - the true name of God - has been hidden under translators' conventions. It is variously referred to as the Mount of the LORD, or the mountain of the LORD, or the hill of the LORD - all are written as *Har Yehovah* in the Hebrew Bible. Therefore, Scriptures like Psalm 24 and Isaiah 2:3 and various others are obscure to the reader who knows not that this is the Mountain of God - Har Yehovah.

"*Come let us go up to Har Yehovah... and we shall walk in His paths. And out of Zion shall go forth the Law, and the Word of the Lord from Jerusalem!*" (Isaiah 2:3). Have not those things already happened? Remember these are end times prophecies. The hidden is coming to light. Other hidden things in the Torah will be revealed. Now that I have recovered, authenticated and begun the translation of *The Hebrew Gospels* the "Word of the Lord" (Yeshua) will be available from the original Hebrew manuscript tradition. There is a massive movement of the Spirit coming. HalleluYAH !

Appendix 4: Bibliography
Red Sea Road to Sinai

Breggin, Peter - *Brain-disabling Treatments in Psychiatry,* Springer Publishing Company, New York (2008)

Breggin, Peter - *Toxic Psychiatry*, St. Martin's Press, New York (1991)

Carnes, Patrick - *Facing the Shadows: Starting Sexual Relationship Recovery*, Gentle Path Press (2015)

Freeman, Rita - *Body Love – Learning to Like our Looks and Ourselves*, Gurze Books (2002)

Hoffman, Natalie - *Is it Me? Making Sense of your Confusing Marriage: A Christian Woman's Guide to Hidden Emotional and Spiritual Abuse*, Flying Free Media, Rosemount MN (2018)

Holm-Denoma, J. M., Witte, T. K., Gordon, K. H., et al.. *Death by suicide among individuals with anorexia as arbiters between competing explanations of the anorexia-suicide link,* **Journal of Affective Disorders**, 107 (1-3), 231-236 (2008)

Holm-Denoma et al - Kaye, 2008 - Keel et al. 2003. American Association of Suicidology.

Jones, Miles - *Moedim: Celestial Events in the Heavens,* Great Publishing Company, Kerrville, Texas (2024)

Keel, P. K., Dorer, D. J., Eddy, K. T., Franko, D., Charatan, D., & Herzog, D. B. - *Predictors of mortality in eating disorders*, **Archives of General Psychiatry**, 60 (2), 179-183. (2003)

Kruse, Jack. HYPOXIA #15: BLUE LIGHT CAUSES IRREVERSIBLE HYPOXIA IN ALL CELLS. https://jackkruse.com/

Lamberg, Lynne - *Interest Surging in Electroconvulsive and Other Brain Stimulation Therapies,* **Journal of the American Medication Association** (JAMA) (September 12, 2007)

Lerner, Harriet - *Women in Therapy*, Harper Collins Publisher, New York (1988)

New King James Version Study Bible, Thomas Nelson, Inc., Nashville, TN (2007)

Peterson, Jillian & James Densley - *The Violence Project*, Abrams Press, New York (2022)

Quinn, Connie. DSW, LCSW-R, Director: The Renfrew Center of New York.

Shrier, Abigail - *Bad Therapy: Why the Kids Aren't Growing Up*, Sentinel Press, an imprint of Penguin Random House, New York (2024)

Townley, Lisa - *Getting Right with God: Exploring Intimacy through Daily Journaling and the Courts of Heaven*, Christian Book Publishing, USA (2018)

Udo, T., Bitley, S., & Grilo, C. M. *Suicide attempts in US adults with DSM-5 eating disorders*, BCM Medicine (2019)

Weaver, Patrick. *The Exodus Project* theexodusproject.com or patrickweaver.org

Appendix 5: Contact Details

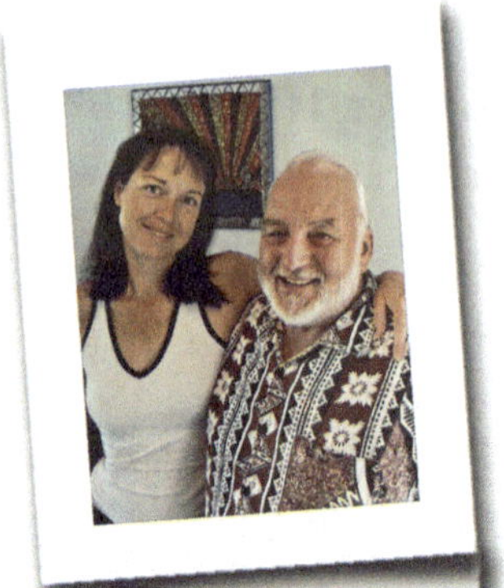

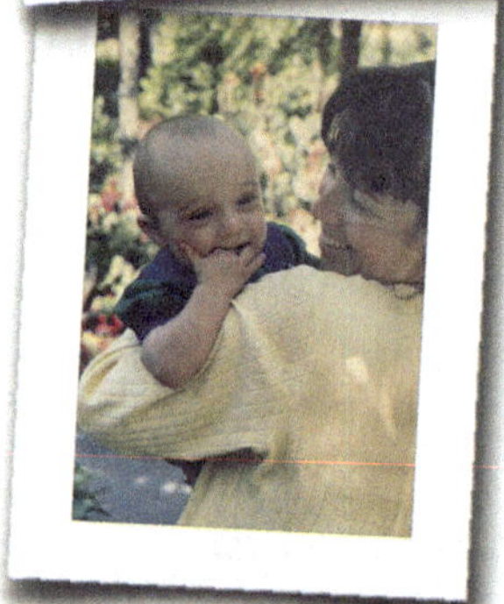

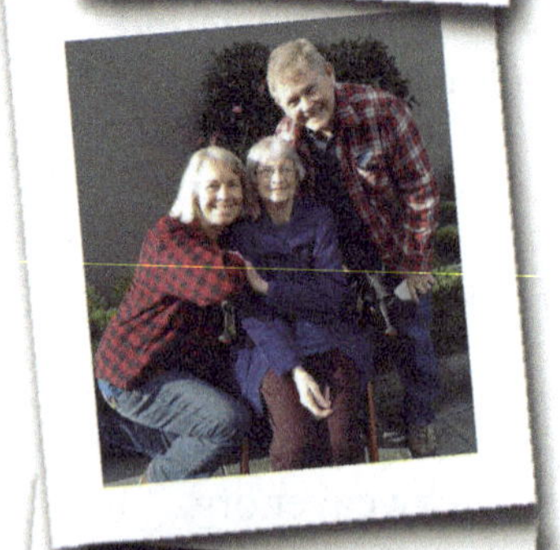

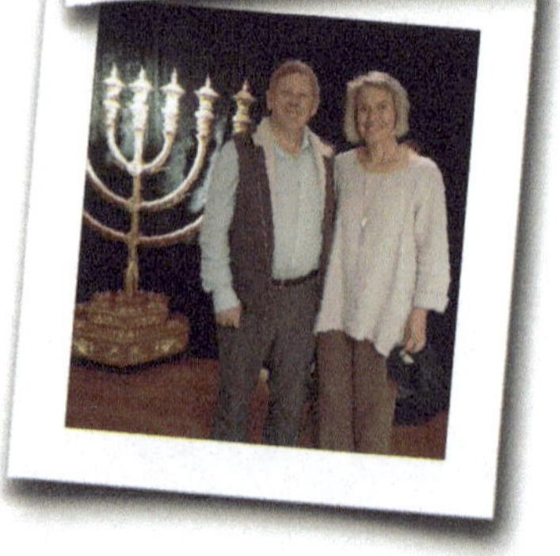

To contact Cate Jones:

Cate Jones
Writing of God
PO BOX 294047
Kerrville,
Texas 78029
USA

Or email:

CateJones@WritingOfGod.com

To see more about this book:

www.RedSeaRoadtoSinai.com

To learn more about the Mt. Sinai expedition and see videos, go to:

WritingOfGod.com

Or to our YouTube channel:
WritingOfGod

**Photos: Cate and Dad,
Cate and Levi,
Cate with Mum and Miles,
Cate and Miles**

Made in United States
North Haven, CT
11 November 2026

22113771R10196